My Ambulance Education
Life and Death on the Streets of the City

Joseph F. Clark

FIREFLY BOOKS

A Firefly Book

Published by Firefly Books Ltd.

Text copyright © 2009 Joseph Clark

First Printing

National Library of Canada Cataloguing in Publication Data

Clark, Joseph F. (Joseph Floyd)
    My ambulance education : life & death on the streets of the city / Joseph F. Clark.
ISBN-13: 978-1-55407-464-8 (bound)   ISBN-10: 1-55407-464-9 (bound)
ISBN-13: 978-1-55407-447-1 (pbk.)   ISBN-10: 1-55407-447-1 (pbk.)
    1. Clark, Joseph F. (Joseph Floyd). 2. Ambulance service — New York
(State) — New York. 3. Emergency medical services — New York (State) —
New York. 4. Emergency medical technicians — New York (State) —
New York — Biography. I. Title.
RA645.6.N7C53 2009   362.18'8092   C2008-907447-5

Publisher Cataloging-in-Publication Data (U.S.)

Clark, Joseph F.
    My ambulance education : life & death on the streets of the city / Joseph F. Clark.
[256] p. : col. photos. ; cm.
Includes index.
Summary: A look inside the intense life of an emergency medical services worker.
ISBN-13: 978-1-55407-464-8   ISBN-10: 1-55407-464-9
ISBN-13: 978-1-55407-447-1 (pbk.)   ISBN-10: 1-55407-447-1 (pbk.)
    1. Clark, Joseph F. 2. Emergency medical technicians — New York (State) —
New York — Biography. 3. Emergency Medical Technicians — Personal
Narratives. 4. Emergency Medical Services — Personal Narratives. I. Title.
362.18097471/092 B dc22   RA645.6.N7.C537   2008

Published in the United States by
Firefly Books (U.S.) Inc.
P.O. Box 1338, Ellicott Station
Buffalo, New York 14205

Published in Canada by
Firefly Books Ltd.
66 Leek Crescent
Richmond Hill, Ontario
L4B 1H1

Text design: Erin Holmes
Cover design: Richard Cote, Sideways Design

Printed in China

The Publisher acknowledges the financial support of the Government of Canada through the Book Publishing Industry Development Program for its publishing activities.

CONTENTS

Foreword 6

Introduction.. 8

1. John Doe and Company 11
2. Introducing Death 21
3. Christmas Eve 29
4. Suicide Is Painful 41
5. Lost Glasses and Drugs to Go........................... 51
6. A Crushing Blow... 63
7. Tunnel Vision 73
8. Bob the New Guy... 81
9. Sleep Depraved 93
10. Vomit on the Ceiling 107
11. Angel Dust 119
12. The Streets.. 137
13. Shake and Bake and Other Ambulance
    Regulars... 147
14. Visiting the Newborns....................................... 159
15. Drunks Are a Part of the Job 167
16. Along for the Ride... 177
17. Brothers in Arms 187
18. Alternate Uses for the Ambulance 197
19. Killing Time in the ER 207
20. Spic and Span.. 217
21. My Ambulance Ride 223
22. Holly Holiday.. 227
23. The Big One.. 231
24. Last Call 239
25. Afterword 247

Glossary 248

About the Author... 251

Picture Credits... 251

Index 252

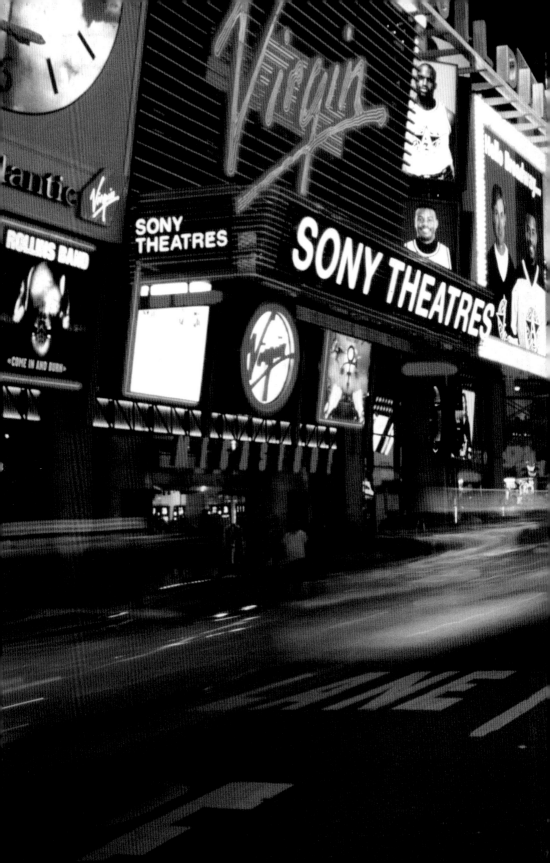

DEDICATION

Working the emergency services is a continuous learning experience. Thus this book is dedicated to all my teachers, especially the two best teachers I ever had:
Mom and Dad

FOREWORD

In this era when terrorism and disasters are very real threats to all of us, we have a new awareness and appreciation for the services provided by emergency medical service (EMS) personnel. Yet for more than 40 years, EMS personnel have toiled diligently to take care of people in their hour of need. One patient at a time, these unsung heroes have placed the interests of others before their own and saved countless lives.

My Ambulance Education by Joseph Clark is a testament to the challenges that EMS personnel everywhere face daily. Whether they are assisting a patient who is having difficulty breathing, treating someone's pain, or merely providing safe transport to the hospital for a psychotic patient, they must always be prepared to help the next person for whom they are summoned. They do this willingly and seldom with any accolades.

Despite the personal rewards that EMS personnel often receive from all of this, their jobs exact an emotional toll—a big one. There is an emotional strain that is often overlooked and rarely discussed for fear that this would be perceived as weakness. *My Ambulance Education* is more than a collection of experiences. It's more than an accumulation of intense life events that most of us will never encounter. It is a daring and open debriefing session, a necessary unburdening of an emotional weight that would crush most of us.

This book's bold approach reaches a balance that many books attempt, but few achieve. It is frightening yet humorous, disheartening yet inspirational. These are just a few of the emotions in the complex mix that our EMS personnel are expected to manage every day. Joe Clark was no exception. Now, his shared experiences offer us a peek into the nonstop challenges of this job. His delivery is natural, genuine and brutally honest.

Prepare yourself for a roller coaster ride of emotions as you enter a world of psychological stress and physical challenge. Some people, such as EMS personnel, will find it liberating to share "war stories" and (finally) openly confess the emotional strain that they, as heroes, have endured for so long. But everyone can learn from the experiences recorded in these pages.

Todd Crocco, MD
Chair, Department of Emergency Medicine
West Virginia University
Morgantown, WV

INTRODUCTION

I started working on an ambulance when I was 18 years old and in high school, and I actually considered making it my career. But I headed to college as a chemistry major instead. This ended up being the ultimate double life, because the student lifestyle is very insular and not an accurate reflection of reality. In college, if you make a mistake in a test there may be a final or makeup so you can do it over. But in life, and on the ambulance, there is no such thing as a do-over. The ambulance life is excessively harsh and contains more reality than most people should have to deal with. When I was faced with the choice of making a career as a paramedic on the ambulance or heading toward another destiny by being a college student, the choice was easy. Today, I am still in college—as a professor.

One of the few harsh realities of being a student is that college costs money. I did not have the money for tuition, and the ambulance was willing to pay me. People need ambulances 24 hours a day, seven days a week. So I could go to classes during the day and work nights and weekends. There was no shortage of shifts, and it meant a steady income to cover college fees. I put in 36 to 48 hours almost every weekend during term, and worked full-time during breaks. Full-time on the ambulance was 60 to 100 hours a week. If things were slow, I could even study while working a night shift. Although I pulled a lot of all-nighters on the ambulance, I never stayed up all night studying for an exam or preparing a paper. Sleep was too valuable to lose because of a test.

I decided to write this book because paramedics and EMTs deserve more recognition for the service they provide to the public and the hospitals they serve. The tragedies of September 11, 2001 highlighted the importance of emergency services. The heroism and dedication seen on that day and in the months that followed were not a surprise to those on the job, but the appreciation and thanks from the public was long overdue. Paramedics receive as many as 3,000 hours of training, enabling them to make early assessments of patients and treat many medical emergencies. They are highly skilled professionals who are able to apply the latest medical research to give every patient the best possible chance of surviving.

I firmly believe that public health would be greatly improved by doing research that leads to better therapies for the patients on the ambulance while they are in the critical first minutes after a life-threatening event. By bringing the emergency room to the ambulance, a paramedic can save lives before patients even get to the hospital. Although I do not plan to work on the ambulance again, the people still on the job have my respect, my sincerest admiration and even my sympathy. We all have defenses that enable us to deal with the job. This book is my ultimate defense system.

The events portrayed in this book are based on fact, though I have changed the names and altered the order of some events. These stories are a distillation of about eight years of working on three ambulances and two emergency rooms in New York and Michigan. These experiences have shaped, and are still shaping, my career as a university professor.

I do not recommend doing what I did to pay university tuition, but neither would I trade the memories for anything.

John Doe and Company

When the holidays are approaching, death always seems to take on an added poignancy. During my first year on the ambulance, fall came and went all too fast and the winter was here. High school kids were learning the skills they would need for life, and one of these skills is driving. Teenagers kill themselves all too often in car accidents caused by speed and reckless driving, but a car can kill in many ways besides the shocking wreck wrapped around a tree.

Tom was a great partner who was my age and quite experienced. He was working on the ambulance full-time to pay for school—as he put it, he was on the eight-year plan, because it was going to take him that long to finish college. Tom wanted to be an engineer and make prosthetic devices for people who lost limbs. He had a slight build and looked frail, but this appearance masked a dynamic and energetic person who could be a powerful one-man army if necessary. It was rumored that he was a third-degree black belt in karate and knew a half dozen ways to kill a person with his bare hands. Tom was not a person to mess with, but I liked him a lot and enjoyed spending time with him both at work and away from it.

One very cold winter morning we were called to the scene of a "person not moving in a car" in the park. I first imagined a drunk who fell asleep and might be hypothermic. We arrived with the cops to find a car and something in the back seat that looked like a person not moving. The doors were locked, so after a bit of pounding on the car to see if someone would wake up, we smashed the windows and let ourselves in. Only then did I realize that the car was running. The inside was warm, with a ripe smell of exhaust and dead person. Two persons to be exact: a teenage boy and girl, both dead from carbon monoxide poisoning. Their arms, legs, lips and lower extremities were locked together in a lasting and terminal embrace.

Apparently they had headed out to the park for a late-night rendezvous to celebrate the victory of the local high school football team. They parked the car, got in the back seat, took off their clothes and got under some blankets. The driver had left the engine and heater on. The problem was that he had backed up into a snow bank. The snow blocked the exhaust, so the car filled with odorless but deadly fumes. They enjoyed a night of passion and fell asleep with their lips joined in a deep kiss. I had to pull their heads apart to check for signs of life and saw that each bore the impression of the other's puckered lips after I separated them.

There was nothing we could do for them, but we nonetheless decided to take them to the hospital by ambulance. Though not completely standard operating procedure (SOP), we occasionally did this to provide the gentlest possible environment for the families—so they could identify the bodies in the ED rather than the morgue. Tom and I started to untangle the arms and legs of these two completely naked lovers, a John and Jane Doe. (Using the terms John and Jane Doe for unknown persons, even in written reports, is common practice in medicine—not just in North America, but around the world.) John was on top, but when we started to lift him off of Jane something prevented us. They were joined at the waist. They had been making love when they died and he was still inside her. I ended their coital encounter that morning and John Doe was shipped off to the hospital with all his anatomy present and accounted for. There is no delicate way to describe the process of retrieving his male organ—this is not a technique they teach ambulance personnel—but it did remind me of an old joke. What did the leper say to the prostitute? Keep the tip.

The story of Jane and John Doe made the papers. Previously, when I participated in calls that made the news, I was generally shocked at how poorly the papers presented the facts of the call. This time, however, I was grateful for how little detail they included about John and Jane's last hours. Tom said the paper should have made it clear that they went out with a bang. Blunt as he was, Tom's defense was humor and this was his way of dealing with the tragic loss of two high school students.

The weather got even colder during the next few days. One of these mornings Tom and I were called to an exclusive neighborhood known for its large single-family houses. The call came in simply as "police request an ambulance," so we had no idea what we would see when we got there. When Tom and I arrived at the address, there were already two police cruisers and an unmarked car in front of the house. The unmarked car was a bad sign, because that meant a police supervisor was needed at the call. We were soon speaking with the detective supervising the scene, who was underdressed for the weather. With his hands firmly in the pockets of his flimsy jacket, he brusquely said, "We have a murder scene. Confirm the corpse is a corpse, don't touch anything, and get out."

It is not uncommon for the PD to request a confirmation of death at the scene, so we were there to make sure the person in question was deceased and let the ME take the case. The odd part of this scene was that the corpse was under the porch of an affluent person's house. The homeowner had found the body and the cops didn't want it moved until they had a chance to see if there was any evidence. I had experience with this sort of thing, so I grabbed a stethoscope as well as a flashlight and headed under the porch. There I found a middle-aged white man with Mediterranean features.

He was dressed only in his underwear and his hands were tied behind his back with duct tape. He was sitting up with his legs apart, propped up by his hands behind his back. His head was leaning forward and there was a bloody icicle hanging down the right side of his face coming from the single bullet hole in his right temple. I placed the stethoscope on his bare back and it made a clinking noise. This gentleman was frozen solid. With my bare finger, I tapped his back and it felt like a frozen chicken right out of the freezer. He was definitely very dead.

I crawled out of the porch and turned the scene over to the police. Tom and I stayed to write up the call and observe the spectacle. There was an impending logistical problem and I wanted to see how the police dealt with it. The entrance to the crawlspace beneath the porch was very low and narrow. The corpse was frozen solid and spread out in such a way that it would be impossible for it to pass through the opening. I wanted to watch as they went through the process of advising the homeowner that they would have to disassemble part of his porch before the body could be removed. We also stayed to see if we could get a name to use in the paperwork. Tom suggested just writing it up as a John Doe, but I said that since we'd already done a John Doe that week we ought to use another name. I suggested Papa Doe, because the victim looked like the stereotypical Italian mafia boss. Tom, however, suggested a better name: Popsicle Doe.

Though the facts behind this call may never be fully known, it appeared that Popsicle Doe was killed as part of a mob hit and the body placed at that address as a message to the residents. (I diligently scanned the obituaries and watched for news stories on this victim, but I don't know if Popsicle Doe was ever identified.) The homeowner denied knowing who Popsicle Doe was, so we filed the report with that name. Before we left though, Tom and I said the paramedic blessing for Popsicle Doe: "He's dead meat. Let's beat feet."

Very late that night, Tom and I entertained ourselves by listening to the police chase a burglar across the rooftops of a block of buildings. The chase ended suddenly and a call went up for the ambulance. We knew it was for the burglar and not the police because the call came in as "police request the ambulance at the scene." If a police officer was injured, they would say "officer down." Those words would mobilize the emergency services, but that was not what we were heading to now. It turned out that two officers were chasing the suspected thief when he tried to jump across an alley to the neighboring building. I'm sure he had seen a bad guy on TV get away by doing this, but this time the bad guy missed the roof he was aiming for. He hit the wall of the brick building and slid down it to the alley below. The fall was seven floors, so he was not likely to survive. When the younger of the two officers saw the guy fall, he turned to run down to the alley. His partner grabbed him and said, "Do you think he is going to get up and run away?" So the two of them walked down the stairs while calling the ambulance.

When we arrived, Tom went to check our patient while I brought the equipment. The burglar was dead, so we needed to determine what the police wanted us to do. This type of scene would require an investigation to ensure that the rights of the burglar had not been not violated. We would probably have to wait for the medical examiner to turn up and release the body to the ME's office. But the cops seemed to be preoccupied with shining their flashlights on the wall of the building and looking intently at it. What was so interesting for them were the obvious bloody streaks: the burglar had left skid marks down the side of the building as he fell. When we looked closer at the body in front of us, we saw that the man's hands and fingers were severely scraped and scratched, with fingernails missing. Our fleeing burglar had clawed the wall like a cat as he fell, eventually losing his battle with gravity. Visions of a Garfield cartoon scene kept popping into my mind. When we got to the point of trying to identify the burglar we found he had no ID on him. I immediately suggested calling him Garfield Doe and the cops and ambulance personnel unanimously agreed.

Tom and I seemed to have bad luck on calls, with more than our share of unidentifiable bodies. It's bad enough when a body (and any paper ID in the wallet or purse) has been burned beyond recognition and dental records must be used. The real problem, however, comes when the severely burned victim is still alive.

Burn victims were always difficult calls. Severe burns—third-degree burns over more than 50 percent of the body—are often lethal and it is difficult to handle the patient without removing skin or tissue. The severely burned patient needs fluids, but the skin covering the veins that we normally would use to provide those fluids has been turned to bacon and gristle. Thus the ambulance crew will usually douse the person with sterile water and get him or her to the hospital, where the patient can be given IV fluids through lines into major vessels.

On one of our worst calls, a Ford Pinto was hit from behind by a delivery truck and both burst into flames. The truck driver was able to get out, but the Pinto driver was trapped. We arrived with the fire department, which quickly put out the flames, but there was little hope of finding anyone alive in the burned-out wreck. Nonetheless, Tom went in to check. Inside was a person with third degree burns over what looked to be his entire body. Since he was still in the seat, we couldn't assess the burns on our patient's back, but his front was as black as a hamburger lost in the coals of a backyard grill. I was waiting for Tom to confirm that John Doe was DOA (making him a "DoDo") so we could leave, when he called me over to the car. I grabbed the trauma box and ran to him. Pale and sweating from the heat of the burned car and cooked victim, Tom exclaimed that the victim was still breathing. This galvanized everyone at the scene into action. Our victim was making loud rasping breaths that seemed to crackle like a freshly poured cola. The unusual breathing noise was caused by the trachea, or windpipe, being burned and swollen, narrowing of the air passage. The crackling noises were likely a result of the tissue in his chest being cooked, and thus unable to move with his breaths.

The heat of the fire was cooking his flesh, so our patient needed to be cooled immediately. The fire department gently hosed him down to cool his body while being careful not to spray water in his face. (Water in the face could be inhaled into the lungs.) Next, we needed to get him out of the car as quickly as possible. But knowing the fragile state his skin would be in after such burns, we would need help in moving him gently.

I called over a couple of firefighters and they quickly got the door off the car. We then tried to slide the crispy critter out of the car and onto the stretcher. Tom and I were pulling him towards us and guiding him onto the stretcher when all of a sudden there was a loud ripping noise and a pop. John Doe's arm came off into Tom's hands. All four emergency services person-nel froze in stunned silence. My stomach was knotted with the horror of what we had just done. As we stared at him holding the left arm of this still-breathing burn victim, he turned to me and gesturing with the charred arm said, "Wanna bite?"

The laughter that followed was forced. Tom was a true believer in the idea that jokes are one of the best defenses against the stresses of this job. None of us really thought his joke was funny, but it jolted us back into action. When we got John Doe on the stretcher, we had to have him sitting up, because all his muscles were cooked into the sitting position. Even his remaining arm was thrust forward as if he was still gripping the steering wheel. As Tom drove us to the hospital and I checked again for breathing sounds coming from our unfortunate passenger. There were none. There was no place on his body where I could easily check for a pulse and because of the position he was stuck in, I couldn't even consider CPR.

We drove to the hospital with lights and sirens as I sat in back looking at the burnt shell of a man that continued to radiate the heat he had absorbed during the fire. I stared blankly and helplessly at the hole where our patient's left arm had been. It oozed a thick, viscous blood that dripped down onto the stretcher and pooled on the floor. I tried not to think about the barbecue smell that dominated the ambulance. When we arrived at the hospital I could see in Tom's red, puffy eyes that he was feeling the anguish of what we had been through.

Later, after we got the greasy feel of burnt human flesh washed off our hands, I asked Tom, "Do you want me to write up this John Doe?"

Tom knew I was really asking him if he was OK, and he came back with the only reply that would tell me that he was. He said, "His name is Barbecue Doe, and I want to write it." He wrote the call up with surgical precision and detail and dealt with the rest of the day's calls with his typical gallows humor, but we avoided talking about Barbecue Doe.

Introducing Death

Police, medical personnel and clergy are all professionals who deal with death regularly. Death is part
of the business. Many people ask me about the worst
or most disgusting call I ever had, and some even ask
about the worst dead body I ever had to deal with during my years on the job. For me, the dead body that
was the hardest to deal with was one of the first I ever
encountered. A person is a person, and when life ends
the body is a bag of cells, proteins, salts and water.
However, that bag of cells was once someone's son,
daughter, husband, wife or loved one. The John and
Jane Does emergency personnel often have to deal with
were loved by someone, somewhere.

Just before sunrise on a clear spring morning, we were
called to assist a police officer. The location was not
an address, but a lonely stretch of road. Roger, the cop,
had observed a car traveling erratically and pulled over

the lone female driver. The woman in her late 40s was dressed in a pink nightgown that made her seem almost ethereal. She stopped and immediately jumped from the car and started to run along the grass verge. Roger ordered her to stop and she appeared to trip and fall face first into the grass. When Roger came up to her she was not moving and apparently unconscious. When he placed his hand on the middle of her back to prevent her from rolling over and turning on him, his hand was pierced by a knife. She hadn't stabbed him—a large knife had been stabbed into her chest so far that the point was sticking out of her back.

When we arrived Tom bandaged the cop's cut hand and I went to see the woman. We were not sure if this was a suicide, accident or homicide, so I had to work carefully to preserve the scene. It was easy to see the knife protruding from the middle of her back, just to the right of her spine. Blood was oozing out around the point of the knife and flowing down her right side; the handle was out of sight underneath her. I couldn't reach her wrists to take a pulse because they were beneath her body as well. Her head was turned to the side, and as I moved the long black hair from her face to try to take a carotid pulse, I got a close look at her. Much to my horror I was looking at the body of Mrs. Collins, the mother of a very close friend of mine from high school.

I had known her son Ryan for many years and been to their house often. I shared dinners there, too. While this changed things for me emotionally, I still needed to work the scene in a professional way. I knew the medical examiner had already been called and that our job was to determine whether the person in front of me, poor Mrs. Collins, was in need of medical care or if she was dead. I quickly and sadly determined that there was no pulse, no respirations or other signs of life from her. The life had been drained from her by the large flow of blood that had gathered below her body in the dirt. The bright red blood was clotting in a smooth, glistening bed below wild violets just starting to bloom.

I turned to Roger, a patient who could still be helped. But Roger refused to be taken to the hospital. He seemed to be behaving as if the scene was his and he was going to work it. Fortunately, a police supervisor arrived and ordered Roger to be taken to the ED. So Tom drove and I sat in the back with the injured cop.

The medical examiner pronounced Mrs. Collins dead and the crime scene forensic people took over. As we headed for the hospital I mentally began plans to attend Mrs. Collins' funeral. I never told Ryan or anyone else in the Collins family that I was at the scene of her death, nor did I tell the people at the scene that I knew Mrs. Collins. Eventually, the family and the forensic guys were able to piece together that Mrs. Collins had committed suicide. It was not clear if she stabbed herself or intentionally fell on the knife. But a note left on the chopping block in her kitchen apologized for her departure from this world. The funeral was very hard to take. The secret knowledge of being at the scene of her death was a tremendous burden that I didn't want to talk about. This made me feel incredibly out of place and I was only able to offer the briefest of condolences to the family because I feared breaking down.

This episode also made me realize the human drama that followed our handling of a body and how many lives are changed by the loss of one life. I had known this in theory, but had always been able to walk away from scenes and calls and forget them. Now I saw firsthand how Ryan and his family changed after Mrs. Collins' body was bundled onto a stretcher. In the months that followed, I was constantly reminded of the call that changed my friend's life. Ryan became very withdrawn and macabre. His friendships, including with me, soured. Eventually the family moved out of town, probably to get away from memories in their house and around town. What had been happy memories were now reminders of what had been lost. By that time, it was hard for me to go to Ryan's house. The pictures of Mrs. Collins on the walls gave me flashbacks to the scene with her face-down in the grass.

One way that emergency personnel deal with a DOA is to see the ironic or humorous side of the scene. But I was completely unprepared for Mrs. Collins' death and the gallows humor that resulted from Roger the cop being stabbed by a dead woman made me feel less than human. I really wish I could have helped Mrs. Collins.

Mrs. Collins death taught me that I had a great deal to learn, and there would be many ways to get that education. I was both an emergency services worker and a college student, and I wanted and needed to be good at both. Fortunately, there were opportunities where both of these interests could be addressed simultaneously. I was taking an anatomy class with the nursing students during the summer, for instance. It was being offered to professional students and was a chance for me to earn college credit while taking a class that would have been difficult to take during my regular chemistry curriculum. Anatomy is a hard class, because there is a lot of information (and some difficult concepts) to be assimilated and there is a great deal of memorization involved. There are hundreds of muscles in a human body and we had to learn them all, as well as where they connected to the bones, the nerves that controlled them and the actions they performed. These concepts were referred to as, "origin, insertion, action, and innervation."

The 40 or so people in the class included nursing students, pre-med students, pre-dental students and me. It was an accelerated class and a lot of work, but my job gave me opportunities to see anatomy in action. A kid fell down some concrete steps onto some glass, for instance. There was a cut on his hand by his thumb, and he claimed he couldn't feel or move it. We had learned in class about the nerves that control the hand and thumb. The recurrent branch of the median nerve is an important nerve to the hand that is in that area very close to the skin and I realized that he may have injured this nerve. While this injury was not life threatening, he did need a surgeon and firsthand observations like these helped me in anatomy class.

One week we were learning about the cardiovascular system and perfusion to different organs. Each organ and tissue is continuously perfused by blood (that is, it has blood flowing through it) and that blood flow increases and decreases as demand changes. The skeletal muscles need more blood flow when we are exercising, the brain needs more blood during activity such as fast or complicated speech, the intestines need more blood flow after a meal and so on. We were given an essay assignment: "Choose your favorite organ and discuss its perfusion at rest and stimulated." We had a week to finish the assignment and had to get our chosen tissues approved in advance. The next day the professor, Dr. Brenda Oaks, asked the class if anyone had decided on their organ yet. One person raised her hand. Dr. Oaks said, "OK, what organ do you want to discuss?"

"The penis," replied the student. There were a few snickers, but not too many—we were paraprofessionals, and the mention of an organ of reproduction was not a big deal.

"OK," said Dr. Oaks, "that is an interesting choice. That is actually a complicated discussion because of the multiple perfusion changes that occur when this organ is stimulated."

"Really?" said the student, "I thought it was the simplest." That brought a lot of laughter from the students.

From the class a male voice called out, "Can I do the penis too? I have a fond attachment to that organ." Dr. Oaks laughed at that.

I resolved to discuss a skeletal muscle in my essay but I did want to meet the student interested in penises. In the hospital café, I saw her in line for lunch. She looked a little like a young Mrs. Collins. I stepped up behind her and casually asked how her essay was going. "I was so embarrassed," she said.

We chatted briefly and I learned that her name was Holly and she was a nursing student interested in working in the emergency room. I told her my story of ambulance work and college chemistry. She smiled, nodded and said that the ambulance sounded interesting and fun. I agreed and I knew that I would be seeing her again.

Christmas Eve

Before I went to work on the ambulance, I thought that hospitals would have fewer patients during the Christmas holidays. People were probably too caught up in family matters and shopping to go to the hospital—the old "I have no time to be sick" mentality. Well, that is far from the way it is. Hospitals are loaded with patients around Christmas because of the stress caused by all of those extra things to do, family feuds and people being forced to break their normal routines. This leads to heart problems, psychological collapses and intestinal distress, all of which overflows into the hospitals. Hospital and emergency personnel are constantly busy with the sick and injured. We had our share of extra work, too. Between the fresh New York snow, all that Christmas cheer and playful kids home from school bringing up Mom's blood pressure, there was a lot of business for the ambulance.

Despite the hassles and pressures of it all, even the most grinchy emergency room person's heart melted when a homeless guy stumbled in asking only to get warm. "Yeah, sure. Who do we bill?" would be the only question.

I was working the day shift on a crisp, clear and cold Christmas Day. My usual partner had requested the day off, so I was teamed with a guy named Warren McCain. We had never met before because it was Warren's first day on the job. He was a bright young fellow with aspirations to join the Fire Department. The ambulance was a common avenue for getting into police and fire departments. The skills gained on the ambulance came in handy in both departments and we were always hiring because our turnover was so high.

We were doing the 3 p.m. to 11 p.m. shift this Christmas, so I spent the morning with my family. My brother Jim, a cop, had worked the midnight to 8 a.m. shift on Christmas Eve. That left us Christmas morning to celebrate. At 2 p.m., my brother went to sleep and I went to work. Everyone in my family seemed to be on the job. My brother-in-law was in the fire department and my mother was on the volunteer ambulance—a Jolly Volly.

Warren seemed to be a pretty smart guy, so I couldn't understand how he got stuck doing Christmas Day. Jim Conner, the supervisor for our district, must have pressured the poor guy at the interview.

"How did they talk you into doing this shift?" I asked when he arrived.

"When Jim said it was essential that I start on Christmas Day, I realized that they were probably stuck covering the shift. Why else would they hire me so quickly? So I moaned something about having to miss Christmas dinner, and how that was an important part of the holiday for me. Then I casually asked if the company would pay for Christmas dinner, and JC said, "yes.""

"Are you telling me we have tonight's dinner on the company?"

"Yes!" said Warren with a smile.

"Excellent." I smiled right back.

We started the shift confident that we were going to be fed well and reimbursed for it. The previous shift had been slow—not too many calls because everyone was opening gifts and preparing for the day's big events. (Either that or they were too hung over to get out of bed.) But about noon it started getting very busy. The roads were jammed with cars full of people headed to see their friends and relatives. The parks were full of kids test-driving the latest in winter fun gear. Fresh snow and families and friends sharing the glow of warm mulled wine were the perfect recipe for a disaster-filled holiday.

Showtime for the ambulance started with a bang. It was a two-car accident with seven people on board. Four of the victims were drunk. The three sober people were all kids. As the old saying goes, "God favors drunks, small children and the cataclysmically stoned." Both drunks and children do tend to fare relatively well in accidents because they bounce. Kids are more flexible than adults and are better protected by their car seats, so they tend to have less severe injuries. Drunks are anaesthetized, so their muscles remain relaxed during an accident and they bounce around freely, usually with little damage. We once found a drunk woman in the trunk of a car after an accident. She was thrown clear through the back seat and into the trunk by the force of the impact and was uninjured, asking for another drink. In this case, of the seven people in two cars only two had minor injuries and needed to go to the hospital.

The patient on our next call was not drunk, and not so lucky. A 55-year-old man was having a heart attack. We went running up to the sixth floor of a project apartment building in the bad part of town, also known as no-man's land, and found an obese man on the floor, not breathing, with the rest of the family standing around looking at him. They were too drunk to be of assistance. Warren and I immediately got down to business and started CPR. We did chest compressions and respirations to keep oxygenated blood flowing to his brain while we packaged the man up for his ride to the hospital. We told the family that the wife could get a ride to the hospital with the police, but found out that she was out visiting friends and delivering gifts. I immediately had nightmare visions of a screaming wife who had left her family happy and healthy on Christmas Day, only to return as a widow. Yes, widow, because there was little hope for this man. Nonetheless we did our best for him.

The emergency room was still jammed from the previous accident and the rest of the city's hectic holiday. The ED staff ran the gamut of procedures to try to save our heart attack victim, but with no success. He was pronounced dead about an hour after we received the call. Warren and I got out of there before the grieving wife arrived. We didn't want to be there if she went into a state we called "staticus princess." (This Latin-sounding condition is a play on words: *staticus* means "prolonged state," and princess indicates a spoiled or privileged female.) A widow or mother in hysterical grief can be scary to see for family and emergency personnel alike.

The next call came in as "wife cannot wake her husband." Frequently you get that with older people, because one of them dies quietly in their sleep. If it were 7 a.m., I would not have been surprised and would have expected to find a deceased spouse in bed. You spend the call supporting the grieving spouse and getting the body out of bed and off to the hospital. The main reason we move the body in these cases is to give the grieving spouse a chance to come to grips with their loss. It also gives them the small consolation that they did all the right things and that we are giving care to their loved one. A lot of what we do is just applying psychological Band-Aids. But it was now 5 p.m., and it was unusual and unnerving to be dispatched to this type of call so late in the day.

When we got there, there was a beautiful 25-year-old blonde, blue-eyed woman waiting for us. Giggling, she said her husband Dave had had too much to drink last night and that she could not wake him.

Giggle, giggle. "He's not supposed to drink, but it *is* Christmas." More giggling as she led us up the stairs of a spacious brownstone. Giggle, giggle. "I let him sleep because he looked so peaceful and downright cute, but I figured he would want to see *some* of Christmas. The day is almost over, so I tried to wake him."

"What?" I said. "How long has he been sleeping?"

Giggle, giggle. "Since last night. He went to bed without dinner because he was drinking all day. He knows he shouldn't do that. It messes up his blood sugar," she said matter-of-factly.

"Oh, no," I groaned. "Do you mean he is a diabetic who was drinking and has not eaten or taken insulin in over 24 hours?"

Giggle, giggle. "Yeah, he should have been taking it, so this morning I injected him with some insulin. He taught me to do that, you know." She said it with pride.

"Please tell me you also gave him some sugar after injecting him," I pleaded.

"No, silly, he was asleep, so how could he eat?"

This was perhaps the worst thing she could have done. The insulin would have caused his blood sugar to fall, and without some additional sugar there would be none in his bloodstream to supply the brain. She had let him sleep because he looked so cute, but that wasn't sleep— that was a coma. I know many diabetic people, and the first thing they *all* do is teach their spouses to make sure that they don't go too long without food as well as insulin. She was probably taught that, but apparently didn't remember to do it for her comatose husband.

Warren and I did what we could for our patient. We transported him to the ED and gave the report to Holly, the new nursing student I had met in anatomy class. I had come to know that Holly was a strong and intelligent young woman who loved her career and her cats.

Dave survived his wife-assisted insulin coma, but with severe brain damage. After that he was just as goofy as his wife. Warren summed it up with, "That is what I call a real airhead."

The only restaurant open in our area that night was a very expensive Chinese place. "What a disappointment," I said sarcastically. Our supervisor didn't give us a spending limit, so off we went to Ho Yen Wa for a Chinese Christmas dinner. I had never gone there before, and when we opened the menus and saw the prices, it was obvious why. The food was great and so was the service because they had almost no other customers and were glad for the business.

I was working with Warren again just three days later. We hadn't even finished the regular checkout of the ambulance at the start of the shift when we got a call—a "psych call." These were always a nightmare. You never knew what you were getting into with a psychotic patient, especially if they were PFN (plain fucking nuts). They were crazy—the calls, that is. Sometimes you got harmless people who thought they were George Washington and were afraid of Benedict Arnold. But other times there were people who thought that voices were telling them to kill all ambulance personnel. I was a little worried about the latter group.

Warren and I prepared ourselves silently while driving to the call. This entailed removing all pens, pencils, scissors and sharp implements that could be taken and used as a weapon. It is a process called "getting soft." Warren went in the back of the ambulance to get out the restraints we might need. We could only use restraints to protect a patient from furthering injuring themselves or other people (such as ambulance personnel!). We had to keep the leather arm and leg restraints in a locked box in the ambulance because people kept stealing them for recreational purposes. They were the same leather restraints you find in sex shops.

We arrived at the address in less than five minutes. It was a funeral home and there were people dressed in black milling around outside. Inside, we were informed, was a woman named Eve who had become inconsolable and eventually violent during her husband's wake. Some of the mourners were injured with cuts and bruises from what must have been a huge struggle. A violent person—whether they are male or female and no matter what size they are—can be extremely strong.

Warren and I walked into the funeral home, leaving the stretcher and restraints at the door. We could hear loud sobs as we entered. On the floor was a smartly dressed, overweight man who looked strangely familiar. Next to him was an empty casket whose contents had spilled onto the floor. The dead man on the floor was our Christmas Day heart attack victim. Eve seemed to appear from nowhere in a flowing black gown, with flowers in her hair and a veil partially covering her face. She seemed to float through the air like a ghost as she headed in Warren's direction, which made me worry that she was going to attack him.

"I know you," she said with her voice trailing as in song. But how could she? She wasn't there when we tried to save her husband. Eve pointed to him and repeated, "I know you." Then I noticed she was looking at Warren's name tag, which read "W. McCain."

"Cain, my son," Eve said with joy. She obviously thought she was the biblical Eve and that Warren McCain was her son Cain. What a psycho.

Cautiously, she turned her attention towards me. She studied my name tag, which read "Joseph," and said, "Do I know you?" There was a long pause as I tried to think of something to say or do.

"Joseph? Are you Joseph? What are you doing here? Where's Mary?"

I couldn't believe this. "I'm here with, um, your son." I said tentatively.

"I'm so glad you're here," she said as she embraced Warren.

"We'll take you away from here, to a friendly place that will help you," I said reassuringly.

We walked her out of the funeral home and had her sit on the stretcher as we applied restraints to her arms and legs.

"Why do I have to be in this?" she asked.

"We are going to take you for a ride in our ambulance," Warren said confidently, "and everyone who rides in the ambulance must ride in the stretcher."

"OK, my son."

"The rules say that everyone must have their seatbelts on, too," I informed Eve. "We want you to be safe. You will be safe with us."

"Yes, thank you, Joseph."

We strapped her in the restraints quickly and proficiently. Then we wheeled her to the ambulance, accompanied by applause from the bruised and battered family.

Eve had a big smile on her face as we lifted her into the rig. Warren said, "Joe, you drive, OK?"

At those words Eve interjected indignantly. "He's not just *Joe*, he's Joseph." Fear surged through me as she tried to sit up in the stretcher. I thought she was going to get violent and we would be forced to get physical. We were so close to getting her to the hospital peacefully and now it was all about to fall apart. However, she simply said, "Let's go, Joseph."

Eve held Warren's hand happily during the ride and seemed to have forgotten the body of her late husband that had tumbled to the floor of the funeral parlor. Half the family followed us to the hospital and the other half finished the funeral. The family was very impressed with Warren and me. Eve had apparently had other violent episodes and usually needed severe restraining and even sedation. They were amazed at how quickly we had calmed and restrained Eve.

"How did you get her to trust you so?" one rather patriarchal family member asked me.

"Years of sensitivity training" I said.

Suicide Is Painful

I don't know what is going through a person's mind when they are preparing to commit suicide. Frequently, I think the answer must be nothing, because they sometimes do the strangest things.

In big cities, people often jump out of tall buildings to commit suicide. I have been unfortunate enough to actually observe a couple of jumpers hit the pavement and it is a shocking experience. The body makes a sickening noise that is somewhere between a splash and a thud—I always called that unique noise a *splud*. When a jumper goes splud, the body actually bounces. Not quite like a rubber ball, but the body definitely rebounds. It's the bounce that gets the biggest response from witnesses, because it can look like the person is trying to get back up off the ground.

The crowd has a big influence on what a jumper does. I have witnessed a small group of people chanting "jump, jump, jump" when a person is perched on a ledge, contemplating the drop in front of him. These chanters actually got other people to join them and their prompting eventually did convince the jumper to step off the ledge. When he jumped, a cheer went up from the crowd that lasted until the splud and the bounce. At that moment, the once boisterous crowd went dead silent. I doubt any of them were ready for what they saw. They suddenly realized what they were doing, what they had participated in and dispersed quickly. People who encourage and witness a jump tend to leave or deny seeing it, while new rubberneckers come to look at the body.

Steve Estes and I were called to a jumper who, after being taunted and beckoned by the crowd, jumped and made a pretty substantial splud. Steve was a former ARP, a Puerto Rican gang member, who got out of the gang and became one of the city's best paramedics. He lived in the neighborhood he was raised in and was considered a local hero, simply because he was a survivor and now a medical man. He loved the neighborhood and hated the gangs and drug dealers that were killing his people. For him, the degradation of the neighborhood was a very personal loss.

Steve and I went through the usual routine with this jumper, who was still alive when we arrived. Normally when treating a jumper we were watched by a crowd. The onlookers in this case, however, did not want to acknowledge what they had witnessed or contributed to, and they had left. We were there alone with the bloody mess on the pavement. I wondered how those chanters felt when they heard their first splud. The head and neck of the jumper were severely damaged, and it was hard to get air in and out of his lungs. A mixture of blood and phlegm came bubbling and foaming out when we tried to use the respirator to pump oxygen into his lungs. He had multiple broken ribs and our chest compressions were producing a lot of grinding of bones and probably doing little to benefit his circulation. Although the odds were against us, we pressed on with our efforts to save him. We worked well together and did everything right, but he died anyway.

As Steve and I worked our way through the rest of that picture-perfect summer evening, we resolved to head to the beach the next morning. One of the perks of working nights in an East Coast city is that there are beautiful sunrises over the Atlantic Ocean. That particular summer I worked almost exclusively nights. During the day, I would often head to the beach and sleep there all day long. I therefore had the world's best tan—or at least the best tan I had ever had. This system of working nights and sleeping on the beach worked very well for the most part. One day, however, I woke up to find the beach completely empty. The reason for this was painfully obvious—it was raining. I was so tired that I hadn't noticed the light, cold rain that was coming down on me and the lifeguards had all sought sanctuary in their little huts as the bathers left the beach. As I gathered up my stuff and headed home, I felt the eyes of the lifeguards on me and could imagine the conclusions they must have jumped to when they saw me sleep through the rain. Maybe they thought I was dead. I wondered if any of them had bothered to check for a pulse.

I was looking forward to a day at the beach now, but still had to focus on the shift and calls at hand. Steve and I were dispatched to a call of "woman choking." We got there to find a woman of about 45 in obvious respiratory distress. She wasn't choking, but she was vigorously coughing, wheezing and sputtering. There was also a distinct chemical smell in the apartment. We got vitals on a Ms. Reichert and gave her some oxygen, while she explained what had happened. She had chronic asthma and used a prescription inhaler whenever she had an asthma attack. Well, this particular attack was severe and she fumbled around in her purse to find her inhaler. She found it and quickly took a big hit from it, inhaling the spray deeply into her lungs. Unfortunately, she had accidentally grabbed her can of pepper spray. This chemical can be lethal when inhaled by an asthma patient.

Ms. Reichert had immediately called 911 and also took her asthma medication. When we got there, her apartment was filled with enough pharmaceuticals and paraphernalia to suggest a person plagued by medical problems. She was in great distress as we took her to the hospital. I drove and Steve took care of Ms. Reichert. He kept her talking to try to prevent her from getting too excited and to keep her mind off of her problem.

After we arrived, Steve told me that Ms. Reichert had recounted her sad life story in the back of the ambulance as the effects of the Mace wore off. Apparently she had not only medical but family problems. She had recently lost her parents, had a sister in California that she never saw and felt all alone. Steve advised the ED staff at the hospital that this woman might be depressed. The ED was very good at treating the immediate physical injuries, but Steve was concerned that they might miss the psychological ones.

The next evening we got a call that came in as "California woman requests ambulance for her sister." The address was the same fifth-floor apartment of Ms. Reichert. When we got to the apartment, the door was locked and there was no answer when we pounded on the door. Steve and I employed an old ambulance trick to get in—we made enough noise in the halls for the neighbors to complain. We told the neighbors to call the building superintendent to bring the keys to let us into the apartment. While waiting, I had a bit of a brainstorm and knocked on the door immediately adjacent to Ms. Reichert's. An older woman opened the door a crack and I asked, "Excuse me, ma'am, but does your balcony happen to be connected to Ms. Reichert's balcony?"

The neighbor said, "Yes, it does. Why?"

I quickly explained our urgent need to get into her neighbor's apartment. She let me in and I rushed to her balcony. It was connected to the neighboring balcony, but there was a thick cinder block wall between the two. I climbed carefully across the small ledge at the edge of the wall onto Ms. Reichert's balcony. Fortunately, the balcony door was open on this pleasant summer evening, and I rushed past a bleeding Ms. Reichert to open the door for Steve.

Steve brought our equipment over to Ms. Reichert, who was sitting at her kitchen table with a pool of blood spreading out in front of her and spilling onto the floor. On the table were some of her medications, which I recognized from the night before, a straight razor, an empty bottle of cheap wine and a bottle of rubbing alcohol. Ms. Reichert had cut her wrist with the razor, and she was confused and lethargic. Her vital signs were consistent with someone who had lost a lot of blood.

"Did you drink *this*?" Steve asked, holding up the wine bottle.

"Yes," murmured Ms. Reichert.

"Did you drink this?" I asked and I held up the rubbing alcohol. I was afraid that she had. Rubbing alcohol is isopropyl alcohol, which is very poisonous. This would bring the call to a true life-and-death emergency. I imagined the damage the rubbing alcohol would be doing to her intestines and liver. Ms. Reichert didn't answer me—she just kind of shook her head. This response was not very reassuring.

"What is this for?" I demanded, still holding the bottle of rubbing alcohol.

"I used it to sterilize the razor," she said.

In preparing to commit suicide, Ms. Reichert had sterilized the razor she was planning to use. Sterilizing a surgical instrument such as a scalpel is normally done to prevent infection. Ms. Reichert obviously didn't want to get an infection from her slashed wrists. This also meant that she didn't want to die from her suicide attempt. We took her to the ED and she survived. This time however, the ED physician did request a psych consult for Ms Reichert.

According to the psychiatrists, Ms. Reichert's attempted suicide was a cry for help. Her intention was not to die, but to bring attention to herself. This was evident not only in her sterilization of the razor, but also in the fact that she had called her sister to tell her of her intention. This is why the call came in from California.

Fortunately, Ms. Reichert had no lasting physical impairments. Other survivors are not so fortunate—an attempted suicide can result in permanent disability. A non-lethal drug overdose, for instance, can permanently damage a person's brain, kidneys or liver. The result is often referred to as being "Quinlaned," after the tragic story of Karen Ann Quinlan, who was in a coma as a result of a drug and alcohol overdose in 1975 until her death 10 years later. In a case like this, a suicide victim is relegated to a life of dependence upon medical personnel, with no chance of a normal life. Therefore, if you ask an ambulance veteran the surest way to commit suicide, you will be inundated with a barrage of suggestions, including standing in front of a train, gassing yourself with carbon monoxide, jumping from a building (above the seventh floor), jumping from a height of greater than eight feet with a rope tied around your neck, or putting a .38-caliber bullet in your mouth. One that usually comes at the top of the list is to use a shotgun to blow your brains out. A shotgun can do an enormous amount of damage too, and if it is pointed anywhere near the head it almost sure to produce lethal injuries. But nothing, not even a shotgun suicide, has a guarantee.

Steve and I got another suicide call that came in as a GSW—a frantic neighbor had heard a shot. We arrived at a single-family house just after the police, who smashed the window in the door and let us in. In the bedroom was a bloody mess. There was a shotgun blood-splatter pattern on the wall above our victim's head and a tear-stained note on the nightstand. But there was no shotgun anywhere in sight. This made me wonder if it could be a murder.

The patient's face had been taken off by the blast— he had no visible chin, tongue or nose. One eye was completely gone and there was something that looked like a strand of spaghetti connected to a liquid-filled marble hanging on the other cheek. There was no place on the neck to get a pulse and I was trying the wrist when a gurgling sound came from the neck. My eyes met Steve's just as I felt a strong and rapid pulse in the shotgun victim's right wrist. This guy was alive—with no face. The gurgling noise was this poor man, a Mr. Ramone, trying to breathe. Steve and I both picked at the remnants of Mr. Ramone's neck, trying to find the opening to the trachea. We found it and Steve slid the airway into it and ventilated directly into his lungs. Next we started two IVs and packed his face in large trauma dressings. One of the rookie police officers was a bit shell-shocked by this scene and he wouldn't get out of our way. So I gave him the two IV bags to hold and asked him to keep them elevated and watch the drip port to make sure there was two drops a second. This made the rookie feel useful and actually helped us a little. Cops, family and bystanders make good IV poles.

We were just getting ready to transfer Mr. Ramone to the stretcher when one of the cops found the shotgun. The force of the blast had sent it all the way across the room and under a dresser. Mr. Ramone must not have had a tight hold on the gun when he pulled the trigger. He also must have clutched the gun too close to his body, so it was not pointing at his brain. He had absolutely no injury to the brain. When Steve and I opened Mr. Ramone's airway and gave him oxygen, we had saved his life. But we had also consigned him to a life of being blind, mute, and permanently disfigured.

Steve gave the report to the ED physician, Dr. Frank. When he finished, Dr. Frank said, "Mr. Ramone must be the world's worst shot to miss from zero feet."

Mr. Ramone had gone to great lengths in his preparations to leave the world that day. He had left a thoughtful and detailed note saying goodbye. He also used the usually infallible shotgun technique to end it all, but he was thwarted by his unfortunate aim, and then by Steve and me. All he wanted to do was die and we wouldn't let him. I hope he understood that we wanted to help him, even though that was against his wishes.

Mr. Ramone, wherever you are, I am sorry to have changed your plans that day.

Lost Glasses and Drugs to Go

I never liked working the day shift. There were too many supervisors, too many people watching. Night shifts, however, were full of mavericks. No one wanted to work with them—or perhaps I should say no one wanted to work with *us*. Night shift workers seemed to fall into one of two categories. There were unbridled heroes who did great good for humankind, and there were losers with whom no one wanted to work. Both groups were similar, however, in that they both wanted to get away with something. The first group wanted to do more than they were normally allowed to do. They were frustrated physician or cop wannabes who wanted to be someone they were not. People in the second group were often incredibly incompetent or lazy. They wanted to do the absolute least they could while still keeping their job. They were hiding from the administration.

Sometimes, however, people were sent to the night shift because they were *being hidden* by the administration. The powers that be seemed to think that a person on permanent nights would do the least amount of harm and cause the fewest hassles—out of sight, out of mind. This is totally incorrect, but the overachievers were more than willing to take up the slack. So a kind of symbiosis would develop between a competent overachiever and an incompetent partner. (This benefit would be lost, however, when the administration scheduled two incompetents together.)

I, on the other hand, had other reasons for opting to work nights. At one point I had enrolled in a paramedic class while at the same time working on the ambulance and taking some college classes. I got to the point where I had to decide: college, paramedic school or the ambulance. I chose to drop out of the paramedic class and continue as a full-time college student working on a bachelor's in chemistry, while working on the ambulance at night to pay for tuition. (Lots of people dropped out of college to become paramedics, but I was known in ambulance circles as the only person to drop out of the paramedic class to go to college.) Plenty of people got sick and had car accidents on weekends and nights, so I always had a job.

Car accidents with injuries were always an adrenaline rush. Auto-body sheet metal has incredible ways of twisting and contorting upon impact. Sadly, it often wrapped itself with unyielding ferocity around not only other cars, tree trunks, and the like, but human flesh. It was all well and good to have ambulance people and equipment at a car accident, but we needed to get the people out of the cars. Preferably in one piece, if they were still alive.

The police and fire departments were experts at cutting up cars. Those guys from the FD are truly a credit to their profession—at least, they looked impressive and had great tools to work with. They had helmets, gloves, boots, goggles and the finest power tools available. Sporting all this safety gear, the fire department personnel would cut a small hole in a smashed-up car in an effort to gain access to a patient. Still wearing all of this heavy safety equipment, they would then turn to me in my short-sleeved shirt and say, "Go on in."

So, with no safety equipment, I would crawl into the twisted wreck to tend to my patient. While it may sound crazy to enter a wrecked car this way, it was necessary because bulky equipment would prevent access. It could also make a quick exit from the car impossible in an emergency.

Picture, if you will, two people in a space the size of about half a refrigerator: one trapped there and frantic to get out, and the other wriggling into this mess for the sake of the first. As I climbed into these cramped and dangerous spaces, I had no idea who the other person was—all I knew was that both our lives were on the line inside that metal tomb. We had to work together with trust and confidence, but did not have the luxury of time to bond with each other.

I usually broke the ice with a little small talk.

"Hi, my name is Joe. How are you doing?"

"OK."

I would want to say, "If you are really OK, then can I go?" But usually I said something like, "That's good."

Now the formalities commenced.

"I'm with the ambulance and you have been in a car accident. We're here to get you out and take care of you."

"What happened?" was often the victim's first question. (It was also the insurance company's first question.)

"You were in an accident," I would inform them again. It was often necessary to repeat this, as peoples' awareness would wax and wane.

"Who are you?" The patient would say with trepidation.

"I'm Joe, from the ambulance." Just once I would have loved to respond with, "I'm the car accident groupie who travels around the country following only the best accidents. You're very lucky, this is a 9.5. You don't get above that number without loss of life, but in your case there is still hope of making it to 9.9."

"Am I OK?"

"Yes, we are doing everything we can for you."

One time we were at the scene of a single-car, single-patient accident. The sole male patient was named Ron Dieble, and he was about 40 years old and very scared.

"How am I going to get out of here?"

"Let me help you."

We were hope brokers. We were in a caring profession. Other caring professions include nurses, doctors, allied health professionals and social workers. People who pursue professions such as these usually say they want to help people. I always wanted to help people too, so I began training in first aid at the age of 13 and completed numerous first aid courses as a youth. I took an EMT class at 17 and became an emergency medical technician less than a year later. I immediately started working on the ambulance, with a view to becoming a paramedic and making a career on the ambulance. My chosen pathway for helping people was to provide care and comfort to the sick and injured when they called an ambulance. This is what I lived for, and that's what I was doing for Ron. If you were in our ambulance there was still hope. No one ever died in my ambulance. No one dies *in* an ambulance because we did not pronounce people dead in the ambulance. People would be pronounced dead in the wreck at the scene or when they got to the hospital. But no one ever died in the ambulance.

My patient did not know this, though. He was just
beginning to come out of the fog and understand that
we were there to help him.

From the darkness outside, a voice boomed.

"What you got in there?"

"A big 6-incher."

"What?"

"A 6-inch laceration across his forehead, broken nose,
OK on airway and bleeding, broken arm, chest is fine.
Below that I can't see." I gave this summary quickly
and professionally. I would have to assess the chest and
abdomen when we got Ron out of the car. Right now I
would focus on head, neck and breathing.

Our extrication of Ron Dieble was relatively simple up
until the point where he said, "I can't see," with just
the right amount of panic in his voice to make me take
him seriously. Loss of vision can mean brain damage
or other hidden head injuries, so I was quite concerned.

"OK, Ron, you took a good hit on the head. We can
take care of you. Sit tight and don't move. I need to get
your head and neck immobilized." I said while searching through the trauma kit for the cervical collar. The
collar would prevent him from further neck injuries.
As I placed it around his head and neck, I got a good
look at the laceration running horizontally across his

forehead. I was familiar with the dermatomes that surgeons follow on a person's skin to minimize scarring.
These are regions where the skin has a grain to it, and
some lacerations can cut along the dermatomes. Ron's
cut looked like it was running along one of these lines
because it was so straight. Too straight.

"Ron," I shouted, "Open your eyes and look at me."

His eyes slowly opened to expose a blank stare. But he
was staring at me nonetheless.

 "Ron," I asked, "do you wear glasses?" My common
sense said to me that the laceration might be caused
by glasses hitting his forehead as his face hit the windshield. So I wanted to find out if he was wearing glasses at the time of the accident. Glasses or frames could
also be imbedded in his eyes or face.

He blinked, brought the hand of his unbroken arm to
his face and said, "I've lost my glasses! You have to
find them—I can't see without them!"

He stared at me with terror at having lost his glasses
while I tried to hide a smile as I realized that he had
not lost his sight.

"Ron," I asked, "is your vision like it would be without
your glasses?"

"Yes," he replied tersely. "I need my glasses to see."

Accident victims can become very emotionally depen-
dent upon personal effects like watches, glasses, stuffed
animals and keys in the first shock-filled minutes after
an accident. So I did feel for him, but my first priority was to get him stabilized and out of the car. I had
formed a strategy for this by scanning the wreck for
routes out. The doors were smashed, the roof was
crushed and the side windows were no good. The front
windshield was also smashed on the driver's side, but it
did look like a possible escape route. We could peel the
broken windshield out and both exit from there. The
safety glass of the windshield had formed a little basket
bubbling out in the shape of Ron's head. Sticking back
into the car from this basket were Ron's glasses.

"Ron," I said, "I found your glasses."

Ron was very happy to get his glasses back, and I
was happy that he wasn't blind. I was also glad that
the glasses appeared to be intact, so they most likely
did not leave pieces in his face or eyes. They were
however the cause of his lacerated forehead and most
likely the broken nose as well. I will never forget
how Ron looked sitting in that wrecked car, with his
Frankenstein forehead and broken nose, sporting those
eyeglasses that matched his injuries perfectly. All
topped with a big smile.

"Ron," I asked, "do you normally have a front tooth
missing?"

Ron had lost one of his front teeth in the accident too, and I found it sitting on the dashboard right below where his glasses were. A front tooth loose on the floor would have been easy to miss amid the shards of broken glass around. The good news for Ron was that the root was intact, so there was a good chance the tooth could be reimplanted.

We bandaged up Ron, packed him into the ambulance and shipped him off to the hospital. I must admit that although I often felt scared and apprehensive while in a wrecked car with a patient, it was also exhilarating and almost fun. It was just me and my patient, and I was the one person in the world who could help him or her. Getting someone out alive is an exhilarating high.

Rick and I were dispatched next to a location along the railroad tracks. The call came in as "man trapped." A PO was already on the scene when we arrived. A plump, elderly gentleman in a security guard uniform was lying on the ground with his left leg trapped under a railroad rail. The ankle was bent in such a way that it was clearly broken. A young couple was standing beside him and comforting him. Rick broke out the trauma kit and I started getting the patient's vitals. There was a normal pulse in the foot, called a distal pulse, and the foot was warm, with good color. This was a good sign, because it meant the blood supply was intact. The patient's name was William Robinson, but he wanted to be called "Hobo Bill." The young woman came up to me and implored us to take good care of Hobo Bill.

"Don't worry, we'll take good care of your friend."

"We're not friends," she said. "Gareth and I just met him tonight. But it's our fault that he got hurt." She looked ruefully at Hobo Bill. "Sorry," she said.

"It's OK, Sweetie. Don't worry about it," said Hobo Bill.

Hobo Bill was a semi-retired employee of the railroad who was working part-time at night as a security guard. The railroad was repairing this stretch of the track and had dropped off a bunch of railroad ties and long metal rails. Apparently the couple had been walking along the pile of rails when Hobo Bill spotted them and advised them to get down, since the rails were not secured and could roll, especially on the uneven ground at the sides of the tracks. The warning was right and timely, because the moment he uttered this warning, the weight of Gareth and his girlfriend, Wendy, caused one of the big rails to roll onto Hobo Bill's ankle. The rail was much too heavy for us to move safely.

We had to wait for the FD to come with some jacks to get the rail off our patient's ankle. Rick and I stabilized Hobo Bill as he consoled the couple for unintentionally getting him hurt. He regaled us with stories of his life on the rails as a conductor. He would often sleep on his trains and this earned him his nickname. In his younger days he would go with the real hobos on overnight trips. He was sad that the railroad company had forced him to retire, and it was only due to some old friends that he was allowed to still work the lines as a security guard. Hobo Bill seemed to swell with pride when talking about his life on the rails and I could see that his ankle was swelling, too. Wendy and Gareth obviously felt bad about the accident and seemed quite relieved when the FD arrived.

Hobo Bill was a pleasant patient and he was gracious to Wendy and Gareth throughout their numerous apologies. We brought Hobo Bill in without incident, and although this was highly irregular, Wendy and Gareth accompanied him all the way. Rick drove while I rode in back with them all. Hobo Bill's major concern was how soon he would be able to get back to work. The rails were his life. I promised to convey that concern to the ER staff. He seemed comforted by this and Hobo Bill thanked us, which I appreciated greatly. We saw Wendy and Gareth as they were leaving the hospital a few hours later. They said that Hobo Bill's family had arrived and were going to take him home. They also said that they would be keeping in touch with him. I hoped they remembered to do this, because Bill would surely appreciate two new friends.

The rest of the night was relatively calm until 5:13 a.m., when we were dispatched to an accident on the interstate. The first police officer had requested ambulance, police and fire backup for three cars and multiple injuries. Despite the hour there was a long line of traffic behind the accident, so the PD told us to enter on the exit ramp and come up the highway the wrong way. Traffic was going to be stopped for a while, so we would not be running into any oncoming cars. On the scene we saw the three cars; one was seriously damaged in the back end, another had a crushed front end and the third was on its side in a gulley on the side of the road. We went to the car with the damage to the front end and the other ambulance went to the car on its side. The PD informed us that the car with rear end damage had had four people in it, and they were all under arrest in the squad cars. None were injured and they were under arrest for drug violations.

Apparently these four guys had decided to enjoy some cocaine while traveling the interstate. A moving car might make them spill some of their precious drug, so stopping in the middle of the center lane of the highway must have seemed logical to them. Our victim was a male driving to work; he had hit the back of the stopped car at high speed. Fortunately, he had his seatbelt on. He was conscious but somewhat disoriented, with a broken leg. He was, in fact, a colleague and friend. Perry Elder was a very senior paramedic who worked in a different region of the city. In the dark, he probably did not see a stopped car with no lights on. Perry recognized us and actually seemed happy to see us. We kept him calm, packaged him up and brought him to the ED. I called the supervisor in charge and told her that Perry would not be making it into work today.

A Crushing Blow

During one two week stretch, we had had a run of serious calls leading to patients being admitted to the terminal ward of the hospital, also known as the "rose garden." We'd had two Quinlans (drug overdoses with alcohol) and four head injuries from car accidents. Anytime there was a spate of such incidents, the staff in the rose garden would start asking the ambulance not to bring any more work for them. A 10-minute call for us for a head injury or drug and alcohol overdose would mean weeks or months of work for them, and years of pain and heartache for the patient and his or her family. During this particular period, there was a growing sense of dread in the ED.

My partner Bill Smith and I, always sensitive to the needs of others, decided it was time to lighten up the atmosphere. Bill's philosophy was "the more serious the situation, the more serious the joke required."

So Bill called in to the ER that we were bringing in "another vegetable for the rose garden," and then sent an EKG strip by radio telemetry. It looked like a ventricular fibrillation, but we had artificially produced the rhythm by tapping on the electrodes. The ER physician on the telemetry came back with a quick reprimand for using the word "vegetable" to describe a patient over the radio.

When we arrived in the ER a minute later, we were met by the staff ready to work a code. But on the stretcher we had zucchini slices, tomatoes, carrots, celery and some dip and cheese, all nicely arranged as if for a buffet. We all enjoyed this little repast and it was fortunate we were not interrupted by any calls. That day was slow; it seemed we really had foreseen the end of the run of new admits to the rose garden.

A while later, we were at the scene of a car accident with one person trapped inside. The driver of this station wagon was unconscious and caught behind the steering wheel, which had collapsed down and backward against his chest. He must have been a carpenter, because the back of the wagon was filled with woodworking equipment. This stuff had shifted forward as he hit the telephone pole and jammed his seat forward. I crawled into the back seat and held traction on the victim's neck. I also took a pulse, monitored his breathing and described the patient's injuries to Bill as I looked him over. I noticed that he had arterial bleeding from his right forearm, so I called to a colleague to hold traction from the outside of the car as I stopped the bleeding.

There is an emergency services saying that all bleeding stops, even if you do not help it stop: that is, it will eventually stop when all of a person's blood is gone or when his heart stops. I didn't want to lose this patient that way, so I placed my hand on the wound and pushed. Next we applied a quick and dirty pressure dressing and the bleeding stopped.

After the pressure dressing was in place, I took over the neck traction and got comfortable. I was doing inline traction, which means holding the head of the victim and keeping his neck and spine perfectly in line. In this way, I became the splint for his neck, and hopefully prevented any further damage to the spinal cord. Next, my patient and I were going to be covered with blankets, and the car was going to be cut from around us. The blankets were to prevent us from being hit with flying glass, and I believe they also served as blinders do for a horse: if you can't see what is happening, you can't get too scared. Well, my patient was unconscious, so I guess the blinders were for me. I was glad to have them.

Shortly after we were covered up, I became aware of a commotion going on outside. The accident had occurred on a main road into the city at the beginning of rush hour on a weekday morning and it was causing a major traffic jam as cars passed one at a time, with lots of rubbernecking from the passing motorists. Later that day, after John Doe (who walked out of the hospital a few weeks later) and I were cut from the station wagon, I heard the rest of the story.

While we were under the blankets, a well-dressed motorist stopped his car and got out to get a closer look. He must have thought that there was a corpse under the blanket.

"Are you a physician?" Bill asked as he approached.

"No."

"Well, what business do you have here?"

"I just want to have a look."

"You need to leave," Bill said as he called over a police officer.

"I don't have to leave. It is a free country and this is public property."

The police officer said, "You are obstructing the work of the emergency services. You are ordered to leave immediately."

"I don't have to. I can stay right here if I want."

The cop softened a bit and said, "You are partly right. You can stay. In fact, you can wait in the back of my police car with these handcuffs on." Then he grabbed the fellow's arm and arrested him. The motorist continued to protest, but the argument was lost. Finally the police officer said, "Look, you will have a great view of the wreck from here and later we can let a judge decide if you have a right to stand here."

I couldn't believe that rubbernecker's behavior. But he did get a great view and a ticket along with a lecture by the judge.

On another shift not long after, Tom and I got a call around 2 a.m. for a "car accident with PI," giving an address along a strip where there are a lot of bars. I immediately assumed that it was an alcohol-induced accident. We arrived to find that the collision was right in front of a very popular bar. The police and fire departments were already there. (Usually the ambulance makes it to these calls before the fire department, but tonight the fire department beat us because they had already been up for another call.)

When we pulled up to the scene, we saw a Mustang that had run into the back of a parked Cadillac Seville. Everyone in the bar had piled into the street and surrounded the car, many laughing, partying and having a great time. The fire department appeared to be doing nothing and called us over to the Mustang. In the front seat there was a male driver and a female passenger. They were both trapped in the car, and her head was caught between his lap and the steering wheel. He was bleeding and she seemed to be choking. The accident had obviously happened because the driver was distracted during fellatio.

Meanwhile, Tom was on the floor of the car on the passenger side making sure that the female patient was breathing and not choking. About now there were calls from the bar party of, "Does she spit or swallow?" I tried to communicate with the driver, but he refused to talk to me. Since he was breathing and in no risk of bleeding to death, I didn't pursue the issue.

The fire department was about to show off for the crowd by using their car-cutting equipment to extricate the victims. The steering wheel of the Mustang had been forced down and backward by the impact of the crash, and the FD was preparing to wrench the steering column up and out away from the couple. I noticed that the driver was a short person—that is, he was not very tall; I was not making a comment on his damaged organ—and I asked the fire department to give me a minute before they started cutting. I reached under the driver's legs (there was not much room), found the lever for moving the seats, and slid the seat back. This immediately freed the two victims, and caused a cheer to go up from the crowd. The cheer was not for me—it was for the woman, who sat up when she was free. When she saw the crowd, she immediately "fainted" and lay motionless. The male patient refused to let me examine him, so I told him to wait in the ambulance as Tom and I got his passenger in the stretcher.

Given the situation, Tom and I felt that the female passenger might be faking her unconsciousness, so we gave her a little test to see. I lifted one of her arms just above her face as if I was taking her pulse, and held it there for a second. Then I let go. When a person is unconscious, their arm will fall onto their face, because they have no muscle control. But if a person is faking, they will frequently move their arm to the side or onto their chest so it misses their face; this is a normal self-defense instinct. This woman did something I had never seen before. When I let go of her arm it stayed there, suspended just above her face. I grabbed her wrist again and put it to her side. I felt confident that she hadn't received a head injury from the steering wheel. The driver, meanwhile, was in the back of the ambulance in a fetal position, still refusing any attention. Tom drove the four of us to the hospital and I called in our passenger patient as being with "no LOC in NAD."

When we got to the hospital the passenger immediately regained consciousness and the driver continued to refuse medical attention. The police tried to get a statement from the driver and when they came out of the conference room they were laughing hysterically. Apparently, the driver had decided not to talk to the police, and was now demanding some treatment. All he needed were a few stitches; the ER physician assured him there was nothing missing. When he checked out, the discharging nurse reminded him that ice would help keep down the swelling.

Tom and I were soon dispatched to a "motorcycle accident with PI." Most motorcycle accidents include PI: they truly are the worst calls. You have several hundred pounds of metal, machine and man (or woman) traveling at a rapid speed. If something goes wrong, the motorcyclist always loses and the mess generally ends up being taken care of by the ambulance personnel. Many motorcycle fatalities can be prevented by wearing a proper helmet. Please let me say to any motorcyclist who does not wear a helmet because it is "your right" and "your life" on the line, remember the people who have to scoop up your brains are seriously affected by your decision.

We often refer to motorcyclists without helmets as organ donors, because after your head is caved in by the impact with a tree, your organs can be transplanted into someone else. Therefore, if you insist on exercising your right to not wear a helmet, be an organ donor. Maybe that should be made into law.

This accident was a motorcycle hit from the side by a car and the chaos at the scene was worse than usual. I don't remember the car or the type of motorcycle, but I remember my patient. He was a large, well-built male in all the best quality leather gear. However, when the car hit him, the leather didn't prevent his lower right leg from being ripped off. Even though this was the most obvious injury, it was not our first concern. Tom and I immediately checked for breathing and pulse, both of which were present. Tom began to secure and immobilize the biker's head and neck while I bandaged the stump of his leg. Tom was starting the first IV when I noticed a cop trying to look busy at the scene, and I felt he needed something to do. I called him over, handed the biker's right boot to him, and said, "Take this to the hospital." He didn't seem to understand until he took the boot from me that the foot was still in it. Even in the dark, I could see all the color drain from his face and I thought he was going to faint.

He did not faint, however, and with a new sense of purpose, got the foot to the hospital. I didn't have time to examine the foot or even pack it in ice, so I just got it to the hospital as quickly as possible via the cop. The biker survived the accident, but did not have his foot reattached because the leg was too seriously damaged, with pieces missing and crushed.

We returned to the hospital to be greeted by the parents of the female passenger who had had her head trapped by the steering wheel in the previous call. Apparently, her boyfriend had told them that he had refused medical attention because he felt that his girlfriend was more seriously injured. He made it clear that I was remiss in my treatment of their daughter: he told them I did nothing for her. The father was irate and demanding to speak to me.

I informed the father that his daughter had decided to fake being unconscious and that I had verified that and treated her accordingly. He insisted that I explain to him how the "arm in the face" test worked. His tone softened as I went through the story, and then he asked me why she would fake being unconscious.

"Well, I believe she was embarrassed," I said, and then hesitated. Tom and I both looked at the boyfriend, who was staring at the bloodstains on his shoes. Obviously the parents were not aware of why the accident occurred. Together, Tom and I explained the scene and how they were trapped, including the behavior of the people from the bar when their daughter was freed from the steering wheel, and how she responded. Without a word, the mother and father turned and walked towards their daughter's room. The boyfriend was limping towards the ER door when the cops, who were still waiting for a statement, intercepted him, and they all walked off to an interview room.

Tom turned to me and asked, "Do you want to go to *that* bar the next time we have a night off?"

Tunnel Vision

New guys on the job have a tendency to focus exclusively on the patient or the injuries at the risk of missing other important things. It is all too easy to run right into traffic to get to a patient or start treating a broken leg without realizing that the patient has stopped breathing. Rookies and probies (new employees still on probation) are especially prone to this phenomenon because the excitement and urgency of the scene occupy their mind to the exclusion of all else. But it can happen to anyone at almost any time. Fortunately, with two people on an ambulance, your partner is your best protection against a mishap due to tunnel vision.

We were once dispatched to a call where a pedestrian had been hit by a car. This is a classic scenario where a crew can be focused on the patient and miss a second victim, a second injury on the first patient, or even get hit by a car while trying to tend to the patient. Rick and I headed to the location, a busy street with several pedestrian crosswalks known as "the shooting gallery" because pedestrians were often hit there. We arrived on scene to find the cops had stopped traffic and there was an adult male in the middle of the street. I could tell he was breathing and conscious because the cop was talking to him while leaning over and writing on a little notepad. Trying to avoid the tunnel vision trap, I took a good look at the location of traffic, the police cars and parked cars. There were no other victims or risks I could see from a visual sweep of the scene.

The victim had a broken right leg that made it look like he had a second knee joint: his lower leg was broken in at least two places. This kind of break is common in pedestrian accidents, as the leg breaks both above and below where the car bumper hit it. Because the lower leg is made of two bones, the tibia and fibula, this means four different breaks and a lot of damage. Our victim had some scrapes on his hands, likely caused when he fell to the ground, but no other obvious problems. I quickly assessed the man's injuries as we approached him and was telling him the usual "we'll take care of you" and "don't try to get up," when he said, "Hi, Joe."

Sometimes people read my name tag, but an injured person almost never does this, so I was taken aback. I came out of my careful assessment to see my best friend from high school, Eric Houseman, looking up at me. He had an apologetic smile on his face, possibly in response to the shocked look I had on mine. Here was a person I'd known for many years and had been confiding in just a few days ago about work, college and my growing friendship with Holly. Eric was two years older than me and had always been a confidant and someone I looked up to. Now we were in a role reversal: I was in control of his immediate future and well-being. I was also shocked because I had been so determined not to have tunnel vision at the scene, yet I had not noticed the face of my friend.

Rick and I splinted Eric's leg and took him to the hospital. Every bump in the road caused him pain, so I asked Rick to keep things slow and steady. I talked to Eric and assured him that I would call his parents as soon as we arrived, and put in a good word for him with the ER personnel. I also apologized for not notic-ing it was him right away. He assured me it was OK, but I remained distressed by my acute case of tunnel vision. To try and make up for it, I checked in on Eric from time to time during the rest of my shift and made sure I talked to his parents when they arrived.

Day turned to night and the types of calls changed to reflect the nocturnal activity in the city. Our next call was for a car down an embankment into a baseball field. We arrived to learn that the car had not run off the road onto the field, but had raced across the field and into the embankment. Inside the car was a lone female driver, no AOB, with multiple fractures and lac-erations. The front end of the car had crumpled into the dirt, mud and grass of the verge. There were many tire tracks on the field, all parallel and all heading to and from the verge. It looked like she had tried multiple times to hit it, each time backing up and then hitting it again.

It turned out she had driven down onto the field earlier in the day to deliver some baseball supplies. By the time she dropped them off it had gotten dark, and she didn't notice that the verge was shallow at one end, where she entered the field, and steep at the other end, where she had crashed. She smashed repeatedly into the steep part of the verge in her attempts to drive off the field. She finally decided she needed a running start, so she got as far away from the verge as possible and rammed into it at speed. The result was a wrecked car and injured woman still not sure why she couldn't drive off that field. Her tunnel vision had her so focused on the steep end that she didn't see that there was an easy way off the verge. We, however, drove our ambulance right onto the field, pulled up next to the wreck and then drove off the field with no problem at all. Rick did have a problem filling out the run sheet.

"We can't call this a car accident," he said.

"Why not?"

"It's not an accident—because it was an intentional," he said with a grin.

Around midnight we got called to a car hitting a tree with multiple injuries. Two ambulances and three police cars were immediately dispatched. We arrived on the scene before anyone else. Rick grabbed the trauma kit and I grabbed the flashlights and we went over to the car. There was a man waving for us to help some family members in the car. He was the driver and was limping but appeared more concerned about his passengers. In the car were two women, his wife and sister-in-law. The wife, sitting in the front seat, was conscious with injuries to both arms, likely caused when she hit the dashboard. She was wearing a seat belt. The sister-in-law was unconscious and crumpled on the floor of the back seat. She was *not* wearing a seat belt, and this may have been a fatal mistake.

As soon as we had assessed the injuries to the victims in the car, a second ambulance arrived as well as a police car. Rick was bandaging the injuries to the sister-in-law and I was getting out the immobilization equipment when I noticed the driver limping towards me. I looked at his leg and noticed that his foot was twisted. He didn't have a twisted ankle: his left foot had made a U-turn and he was walking on his ankle bone. He was so agitated by the accident that he didn't seem to notice that he had broken and dislocated his ankle. I hadn't noticed either, until now. He was not as seriously injured as the two women were, so Rick and I were treating the right people. However, this was yet another example of tunnel vision. I briefed the arriving ambulance on the injuries of the three victims and we took care of them.

"Man hit by truck" was how the next call came in. The address was the interstate—which was very bad.

A pedestrian being hit by a truck going 60-plus miles per hour on an interstate could not result in anything good. I knew our patient was going to be a mess. Two ambulances, three police cars and a fire truck were dispatched.

We could see the scene from about a mile away. The cops were there and we were the first ambulance. We pulled up behind the truck and the victim was on the road covered with a blood-stained sheet. I thought we were going to attend to the victim, but our patient was not the person on the road, it was the truck driver who was still in the cab. A police officer told us that that the victim was deceased and that the driver was shaken up and needed attention. I'd been so focused on the victim in front of us on the ground that I hadn't given a thought to the truck driver. I suddenly noticed the extensive damage to the front of the truck. It was a large Mack truck with a flat front, and the grille was badly damaged and splattered with flesh and blood. What was most striking about this scene was the imprint of a head and shoulders in the front windshield. As we approached, it became clear that there was flesh and hair in the glass. It was almost impossible not to focus on the disturbing amount of face still stuck in that windshield. Fixated on the gruesome sight, I was thrust back to the reality of our living patient when Rick started talking to the truck driver.

He had been injured by the flying glass that had show-ered the cab when the victim hit the windshield. He was also deeply upset by what had transpired, as he recounted how all of a sudden "this guy" ran into traffic right at him. The man was smiling and appeared happy right up to the moment his face hit the windshield. Indeed, he had jumped head first right into the oncoming truck. It was obvious from the description that the man had committed suicide. His death had a devastating effect, however, not only on whoever he left behind in his own life, but on the unfortunate truck driver. I wanted to help this man, but his injuries needed more than bandages. He needed help I couldn't provide. I felt pain for an innocent victim of a suicide. I wanted to be mad at the guy on the road, but he was dead and that was a tragedy, too. So Rick and I bandaged up the driver, tried to comfort him, and prepared to take him to the hospital.

As we were bringing the driver to our ambulance, I noticed to my consternation that the second ambulance was already loading the body of the suicide victim into their vehicle. I realized I'd had tunnel vision now three times on one shift—that must be some kind of record.

Tunnel vision can be like putting your head in the sand, and on this call it was protecting me from taking in the full scope of the tragedy. Unfortunately, it went further than the two victims and their families. We learned later that a psychiatrist had discharged the suicide victim from a psychiatric hospital—declaring him *not* suicidal—less than two hours prior to the incident. The story of the recently-declared-sane person immediately committing suicide in such a dramatic way was made very public within hours.

Tunnel vision is not all bad, however. There are times where one absolutely must focus on one thing and tune out the rest. For example, at a multiple casualty incident (MCI, or "the Big One" as emergency personnel call it), tunnel vision enables you to focus on one patient and not the morass of injured around you. If you allowed yourself to think about all that was going on around you, you would suffer task overload and you'd quickly become ineffective. You wouldn't be able to help anyone. The trick, then, is learning when to put the blinders on and when to take them off.

Bob the New Guy

New York is a great place to gain experience—notoriously busy, lots of action all the time. I had been on the job for several years and been given the job of training a new partner named Bob. New guys had lots of nicknames, like probies, newbies and FNGs (fucking new guys). It had taken two weeks of night shifts to break in this particular new guy. Nights were the best times to break them in: their mistakes and sometimes glaring incompetence were easier to cover in the darkness.

Bob was a very big and heavy guy with a pale, freckle-faced complexion and the reddest red hair I'd ever seen—it looked like he was bleeding hair out of his scalp. For some reason, when he was in his civvies he always wore green shirts and sweaters that clashed with his hair. Bob was a quick learner, though. He had finished the training program for emergency medical technicians with low marks, but still wanted to work on an ambulance and continue on to become a paramedic. If he had had higher marks he would have gone to a nicer neighborhood. But this was the heart of the city. This place was so full of guns that we called the police station the DMZ (demilitarized zone).

You can always rely on a new guy to bring up all those nifty facts that they make you memorize in school, like that brain damage can start within one minute of a person suffering cardiac arrest. While this is an important fact, we will be working hard to save the victim at 59 seconds as well as 61 seconds. Another thing he reminded me of was that there are seven layers of skin. I, however, am not going to pull on someone's cut wrists to count how many layers of skin have been penetrated. I generally operated on the assumption that a laceration had four layers to cut into: Skin, fat, muscle and bone.

Bob the new guy was very informative and surprisingly competent despite those low grades in the EMT course. He was also very gung-ho. While diligently listening to the radio, he would hear another ambulance getting a call and he would want to take it if we were closer to the address. This is called jumping a call, and it's a major no-no. First, it means more work for us. Second, he would want to do this even when the call was a no-brainer. If you are going to jump a call, pick an interesting one.

There are only two people on an ambulance crew, so you had to have confidence in your partner.

Fortunately, Bob did well with the patients. He could tie
more knots in a bandage than emergency room nurses
had scissors. That made life easier for me, because I
left him with the patient most of the time while I drove.
It's true that, being the new guy, he could have killed
our patient. But someone in control of three tons of
ambulance going 60 mph down city streets can kill a
carload of people, not to mention the ambulance crew.

It was the beginning of my third shift with Bob, and
one of the emergency room staff was having a party
to celebrate a promotion. We stopped by the party to
get some free food—no drinks while on duty. All the
cops and emergency staff would socialize and hang out
together, since normal people would not put up with
us. You simply cannot have a conversation with someone who is "on the job" without hearing about blood,
guts, vomit or death. Which is probably why we were
not usually invited to other peoples' parties.

Only five minutes after arriving at the party and before
getting any food, we got a call. All other units were
out and the call was in the center of our region, not
far from the hospital. We didn't get any details on
the type of problem. The dispatcher only said, "officer requests an ambulance for an injured man." We
went up there 10-17 (as fast as possible, with lights
and sirens) and met two police cars at the scene. This
was a bad sign, because if they felt they needed extra
help, it usually meant a violent or seriously injured
patient—or a slow night for the PD. As we pulled up
in front of the apartment building, a cop came running

out and breathlessly summarized the situation: "Man… hand… severed…"

A totally severed hand is not something an emergency service worker encounters every day. Hanging by a thread, yes—that happens a lot. I have seen some very big "threads," including some that looked more like an arm with a bad cut. Such exaggerations by bystanders were common. But I was made nervous by the cop's description of the hand as "severed." Bob, however, was ready to save the whole world. Out of the ambulance went 250 pounds of new guy—but with no equipment. He was followed by the cop, who began directing the new guy to our patient and our patient's hand.

Being older and slower, it fell upon me to bring the necessary equipment: the trauma kit, a specialized first aid kit for just such an adventure. For a heart attack, I would have brought our medical kit. To the untrained eye, the trauma kit and medical kit may look much the same, but to the professional there is a big difference. When we use the medical kit, which has medications and drugs, it costs big bucks. The trauma kit just contains lots of bandages in various sizes. By the time I got inside with the low-budget kit, the new guy had already taken control of the scene and assessed the situation by saying, "My God, what happened?"

Our patient looked like a Jackson Pollock painting. He was a heavyset white male dressed in bright white overalls, with shocking bright red splatters all over his body and topped by neatly coiffed blonde hair and sky blue eyes. He was standing in the middle of the room holding his arm in the air—*sans* hand. Nothing was hanging on by a thread. Bob, always the professional, informed me that the hand was in the trash. That seemed about right for the surreal scene in front of us.

The victim was a maintenance man, and his hand was severed at the wrist while he was loading trash into the compactor. The maintenance man's name was also Bob. So Bob the new guy took care of Bob the maintenance guy while I searched the trash for the missing hand. I had searched toilets for aborted fetuses, scanned the highway for lost fingers and toes and scoured car interiors for stray teeth, but after years of ambulance work, rummaging through freshly compacted trash in search of a severed hand was a new one for me.

There was a large collection of cheap wine bottles, lots of newspaper, fish heads, fish guts, soiled diapers, at least a dozen tampons and too many sanitary napkins, but no hand or fingers. Undaunted, I dug further. Two fingers finally came into view amongst what looked like a large blob of fish guts partially wrapped in newspaper. With a gloved hand, I tugged the ashen gray fingers toward me—and the fish guts moved with them. They weren't fish guts, they were long, stringy bits of muscle and tendon dangling from what was left of four fingers. The length of the sinews suggested that they came from well up the arm. As the trash compactor's massive piston came down on Bob's trapped hand, he must have pulled fiercely to get out of its grip. So forceful were his frantic pulls that he severed the muscles and tendons before the compactor pulled his hand off. With the skill and care of a surgeon, I peeled off the pages of newspaper from the spaghetti, packed the hand in sterile saline and put it in ice. I then gave the whole mess to one of the cops with instructions for the emergency room staff. Cop and hand were off to the ER.

My next concern was the two Bobs. Bob the new guy had Bob the maintenance guy all bandaged and in the stretcher. The wounded stump was elevated to prevent further blood loss and our patient was sitting up comfortably. But something was wrong. I had pulled out four fingers, but no thumb. It did not take a great knowledge of anatomy to see that something was missing from Bob the maintenance guy's bandaged stump.

I pointed to the stump and quietly asked Bob the new guy, "Is his thumb in there?"

"No. Wasn't it with the hand?"

"Shit."

I awkwardly turned to Bob the maintenance guy, who was dutifully elevating what remained of his limb. "Excuse me, sir, but before this, did you have a thumb?"

"Are you kidding? Before this I had a whole fucking hand!" he said, as he waved his bloody and bandaged stump at me.

I told Bob the new guy to get our patient into the ambulance with the help of the remaining cop and shout for me when he was ready. I went back to look for the missing thumb. Time was now crucial. The hand had been severely damaged by the compactor, and hope of reattachment was fading. I tried to recreate the accident in my mind as I searched the trash. This time I avoided the allure of bloody tampons and focused on fishier things. But no luck in retrieving a thumb. Then I reasoned that if I had my hand stuck in a trash com-pactor I would try to pull it out very forcefully. If the thumb was still attached to the arm—say, by a thread— as the maintenance guy pulled his arm free, the thumb could have been flung a good distance. Sure enough, I found the thumb across the room, on the floor next to a broken dishwasher.

Just then, Bob the new guy started yelling for me. Ignoring proper medical procedure, I picked the thumb up off of the floor and shoved it in my pocket. Both Bobs were in the back of the ambulance looking equally pale as I hopped into the driver's seat for the short drive to the hospital. "Any luck?" Bob the new guy asked. I responded with, "Everything is in hand." I then radioed this simple message to the hospital, "We are en route with the rest of that patient from South Parks apartments." The hospital didn't bother to respond and I didn't blame them.

When we arrived in the ER, the surgical team was gowned and gloved, hovering around four digits and gently peeling pieces of newspaper loose from a spiderweb of tendons and muscles. Everyone was using the utmost care to maintain sterility to prevent infection. They were working like a well-oiled machine to save our maintenance man's hand, ignoring us even though we had the rightful owner of the hand with us. They didn't give me a second look until I said, "Are you guys missing something?"

All I got were blank looks. When I dropped the thumb in the middle of their sterile prep I was suddenly very popular: now their inventory added up. I walked away, deaf to their shouts and reprimands for my unorthodox transport of the missing digit. (Bob the maintenance guy did end up having his hand and thumb reattached.)

Bob the new guy and I went back to the party to boast of our accomplishments. I ate a large bowl of cold chili as my partner told everyone how he did all the work. My friend Steve asked me later that night if I had bothered to get out of the ambulance. "I drove," is all I said.

Bob the new guy and I worked together again the very next day. We were working 3 p.m. to 11 p.m., or second shift. Second shift can be problematic, because it includes the dreaded 5 p.m. rush hour, when all the lights and sirens in the world mean nothing to the slow-moving traffic. At 5:27, Bob and I got a call of "man down" in the park. Traffic was a nightmare, so it took a while to get there. I knew that the trip to the hospital after the pick-up would be worse, so I hoped for a simple knock-on-the-nut type of call. Anything that would need urgent treatment would be bad news.

We arrived to find an elderly man with severely slurred speech and pupils that were unequal and sluggish to respond to stimuli. His right arm flailed wildly when he talked and he couldn't move his left arm. Witnesses said he was walking around unassisted and then just fell to the ground in this condition. The diagnosis was easy: it was a stroke. There was a blockage in one of the arteries to his brain, and he needed blood flow *now*. We could do very little for him, however, except to "swoop and scoop." We got him to the emergency room immediately.

I sat with our patient, Fritz Miller, and monitored his vital signs on the long ride to the hospital. Bob drove this time, because the heavy traffic made speeding impossible and I was concerned that Fritz might crash (which means blood pressure and respirations suddenly decreasing or stopping) and need me to keep him alive. We had him on oxygen, but oxygen to his lungs was of little use—what he needed was oxygen to his brain. He needed blood to critical parts of his brain and all I could do was hold his hand as we made our slow way to the ER. This type of call was known as a "hand job," because that was all I could really do for Fritz.

He did have periods where he seemed lucid. So when he was with it, we made small talk. He had a very weathered-looking tattoo on his right arm and I asked him what it was.

"It's a football crest," he said.

"What's a football crest?"

"Oh, sorry—soccer. It is the crest of my favorite soccer team from when I was a kid."

Now that Fritz was speaking more clearly, I noticed that he had a German accent.

"When did you get the tattoo?"

"When I was eight, after the team won the championship."

"Eight?"

"Yeah, and boy, were my parents mad. You could not remove these things in those days, so I have had this for 83 years."

"Wow!'

"The football club does not exist anymore, though. Even the town where I grew up is no longer. The whole town was lost during the war, and many of our friends and relatives were killed then."

"How did you survive?"

"We escaped to America, changed our name from Muller to Miller and hid our German heritage. I had to tell people the tattoo was a family crest or other convenient lies. I loved that team and my family made me hide it and hide my German ancestry," Fritz said ruefully.

Those were the last words Mr. Muller said. He lapsed into a coma and died while I held his hand. Of course, I told Bob to radio the hospital that we were bringing in a cardiac arrest and worked hard to try to keep Fritz alive, but with no success. His brain was dying and I was powerless to help. I wanted to ask him the name of the town he came from and the name of the soccer team. Why couldn't I give him something to save his brain? I was incredibly frustrated. Fritz needed a definitive diagnosis and quick treatment. My hands were tied and I didn't like the feeling.

That call marked a turning point in my career. It started me thinking that I might be more effective at helping people like Fritz Muller if I were better trained—possibly trained as a physician. Maybe medical school was the way for me. I was a chemistry major in a college class full of pre-med students and I could run rings around them because I was on the job and had medical experience that they did not. Medical school meant a lot more college, but it would enable me to help lots of people in a way that a paramedic never could.

The university guidance counselors were surprised when I went to the office to announce my decision to change to pre-med—surprised because they'd assumed I was pre-med already! I hesitated at joining the cut-throat ranks of the pre-med students because this was not really my style. But maybe those competitive pre-med people were not so bad after all—maybe they really wanted to help people, too.

Sleep Depraved

The ambulance garage was a safe haven for the police department. During some of the day shifts, while we were doing paperwork and stocking the ambulance, up to half a dozen police officers would use the night-shift bunks intended for the ambulance crews. While doing my paperwork, I would have the officers' radios lined up on the desk in front of me. If a call came in, I would key the mike (without saying anything, so the police dispatcher wouldn't know that I had taken the call), write down the information and then go wake up the officer. If dispatch needed to talk to the officer and wondered about the delay in responding, the cop said he or she had been in a "dead zone." Dead zones are areas of poor radio reception.

This arrangement was so popular that one of the senior officers had to drop out of the sleeping circle— his wife had complained that he was sleeping so much during the day that he couldn't sleep at night. She worried that the stress of his job had made him into an insomniac and was so concerned she made an appointment for him with the police department doctor. Obviously, the officer couldn't tell his wife or the doctor that he was sleeping too much on the job. He had to stay awake for a couple of shifts and sleep through the night a few times to quell his wife's concerns. His partner was less than happy with this, because if one was awake, both would have to stay awake. It meant they both had to actually work and patrol the streets. Tough job.

The ambulance crews were allowed to sleep if there were no calls. Nonetheless, we covered the police officers and they covered for us. We were all on the job together and we backed each other up whenever necessary.

One time I was scheduled to work 24 hours straight, two 12-hour shifts from 7 p.m. Saturday to 7 p.m. Sunday. And since I had nothing better to do (like sleep), I accepted an offer to work yet another 12-hour shift. That decision was made easy when my replacement didn't show up for work. A one-person ambulance is not much good, so I stayed on for a third 12-hour shift making it a 36-hour day: Saturday though to Monday.

Fortunately my partner for the shift number three was Bill Smith, a seasoned ambulance veteran. He was also a real expert on oldies music and he had a portable tape player that we brought on the ambulance to keep us entertained on the calls. We weren't allowed a tape player, which made it all the more exciting.

Bill was also able to do impressions of all Three Stooges. Most people can do Curly's "nyuck, nyuck, nyuck," and many can do Moe's "What are you—a wise guy?" But Bill was the only person I ever met who could do a convincing Larry. Bill also looked like Elvis Presley and could do an impression of him as well. If I handed Bill a piece of equipment on a call, he would often respond with an Elvis-like "thank you very much," and then follow that with "nyuck, nyuck, nyuck."

Bill had the wisdom of years of experience on the ambulance. He had seen many changes over that time. He was also something of an ambulance psychologist, in that he had a way of using humor to help people deal with difficult calls. His philosophy was that if you don't laugh about it now, you will be traumatized by it later. If he got you laughing after a bad call, he was fond of saying, "cancel that order of stress disorder." I always got a kick out of this psychological therapy coming from an Elvis lookalike who laughed like Curly.

Bill also seemed to know if someone was compartmentalizing the job. This is when a person handles the work as something completely separate from their real life. They are detached from the call and what is going on around them. If this was their coping mechanism, Bill knew that they would not want to talk or laugh about the bad calls. It was as if the calls did not exist for them. I did this to a certain extent, because I would go back to college and largely pretend that the ambulance life I led did not occur.

On the job, however, I definitely used gallows humor as a coping mechanism. The trick is to not get too sick or inappropriate. Bill had that skill and I loved to learn his art. Other people would lean on religion to cope. After viewing a grisly scene, declaring that "God works in mysterious ways" seemed to provide comfort to some ambulance personnel. Occasionally people would turn to drink to deal with the everyday tragedies we encountered. This kind of behavior had the risk of becoming destructive and it made relationships strained and difficult. There was an unspoken, unwritten rule on the ambulance that no one was ever chastised for their coping mechanism, no matter what it might be. So no matter how sick the joke, you didn't reprimand a colleague for it.

I didn't delude myself into thinking I might get any sleep on this 36-hour shift, especially on Saturday night. The coffee and tunes started right away and the night was hard and fast. We were on the run all night long. I started many cups of coffee on that shift, but I never finished any.

The night began with a black gang member who got caught on the wrong street by three members of a rival gang. Two of them held him down as the third carved their gang's initials in his chest. This was an intimidation technique known as tattooing. Sometimes it was done on the face, with very obvious effects. In this case there were only a couple of courtesy marks made on the face and the tattoo on the chest. Our tattooed friend got a ride to the ER and a surgical resident spent several hours suturing him up. The patient, called Pinto, kept swearing that he would "kill the mothers" that got him. When the cops came to take a statement, however, Pinto had no recollection of who cut him. No surprise there. These guys never talked to the police.

When we brought Pinto into the hospital, I stocked up on latex gloves because we were completely out. Gloves and other protective supplies are essential to prevent us from contracting blood-borne diseases such as AIDS and hepatitis. Bill had been on the job back in the day when gloves were made of rubber and pretty much only used to deliver babies. Bill said that back then you would wear the gloves so the mother or baby wouldn't be infected by germs on your hands. He started work when AIDS was known as a gay man's disease. The mode of transmission was completely unknown. The mindset must have been a lot like during the Black Death. People were terrified of patients with the plague, but there was no good test for it and no one knew how it was spread. That must have been real scary.

Bill often told the story of a black gang member purported to have AIDS (this was about 1979, when we still called this condition "gay man's cancer") who was stabbed in the police lock-up. The cops didn't try to stop the bleeding until the ambulance arrived. The first ambulance was a Jolly Volly that would not touch this "infected" patient. Bill was on the next crew to arrive. The local hospital would not take the victim, who was losing a lot of blood and Bill and his partner were forced to take the victim to a hospital about 10 miles away.

"Those were the good old days, weren't they?" I said sarcastically.

As we brought in other patients that night, we watched the progress of Pinto in the suture room, peeking into the "sewing circle" each time we passed. In the end, Pinto refused to have any bandages on his face or chest, and he walked out of the ER in the early hours of Sunday morning, still vowing to get his revenge on the guys who tattooed him.

When he finished suturing, the surgeon commented that he wished that he'd taken before and after pictures to demonstrate the quality of his work. Surgeons aren't always quite this egotistical. But it takes a very special personality to endure 10 years of medical training—four years of medical school and at least six years of surgical training—to cut into human bodies for a career.

When I say I am going to kill an opponent, it means I'll beat you at backgammon by a large margin. Kill for Pinto meant a meat wagon ride to the morgue for someone. His determination to get revenge put us on alert for impending gang rumbles during the next few days.

We had to be careful when we brought gang members into the ER, so we had a code to communicate this information to the hospital. This was necessary to prevent rival gangs from fighting in the ER. If the other gangs knew a lone rival was in the hospital, they might send some of of their members to finish the job. We called Pinto in to the ER on the radio under the code name "Homme." The emergency service people used three major codes to designate gang members. Along with Homme (the word for black gang members), there were the WTs and the ARPs. WTs (white trash) were the white gang members and ARPs were Puerto Rican gang members, though the term was often applied to members of any Hispanic gang. (I didn't make up the code, so I can't even tell you what ARP stood for.) Not a very politically correct system, but it served its purpose in allowing us to communicate with the ER.

Communicating with the ER was all-important, but we couldn't say too much on the radio, because people were always listening in. Not only gang members, but even newspaper reporters monitored those frequencies and would converge on the ER if they heard something interesting had gone down. Abbreviations and EMS jargon helped us to stay out of trouble. If we were to say that someone was drunk, this could be considered slanderous or malicious. So they were AOB (alcohol on breath). We could not say on the radio that we were bringing in a drug addict, but we could "transport a known subab."

Useful as they were, sometimes these codes and abbreviations went to extremes. One time, I called into the ER on the radio with the following message: "LOL in NAD, with KON, no LOC or SOB, ETA three." This meant: "Little old lady in no apparent distress because of a knock on the nut, has no loss of consciousness or shortness of breath; our estimated time of arrival is three minutes."

We got a call after midnight with another abbreviation: "Man down with GSW." GSW is a gunshot wound. So off we went to no-man's land, the gray border between white and black gang territory. This is where we had picked up Pinto earlier that night. And this is where we recovered Pinto's body now—gun still in hand with a half a clip gone. Pinto had tried to reap revenge, but missed. His opponents, however, did not: Pinto had 12 entrance wounds and 12 exit wounds—two dozen holes in his body.

We did what we could for Pinto. We worked him up quickly and efficiently. From the time we started CPR to the time we turned him over to the ER staff it was only eight minutes and 45 seconds. (I timed all codes using the stopwatch function of my wristwatch.) When we arrived in the ER the full trauma team was there. This code was loud and exciting. They "cracked" Pintos freshly tattooed chest—that is, they cut through his ribs with a bone saw—and tried to restart his heart directly, but there was no blood for the heart to pump.

Especially on the night shifts, the ambulance staff often stayed and worked the codes we brought in. Bill, who was doing CPR on Pinto, didn't even get a chance to be spelled from his compressions before Pinto's chest was open and direct heart massage started. Despite our best efforts, Pinto didn't make it. The surgeon who did the suturing on Pinto earlier in the evening was back in to show people his handiwork, and to admonish Pinto for wasting all that good suturing by getting himself killed.

Things were over for Pinto, but not for Bill and me. Our last call came at 6:45 a.m., 15 minutes before I was to end my 36-hour shift, and I needed to get some sleep. Off we went to a call that came in as "woman can't wake her husband." We knew this meant some poor guy had died in his sleep.

When Bill and I arrived at the house, we found a mature woman sitting on the bed with her ashen-faced husband on her lap as she rubbed his chest. She informed us she was doing "heart massage." I complimented her on her quick action and began CPR on her husband. Bill drove us to the hospital because I was too tired to drive. We brought our patient into the ER and into the same room where Pinto had died a short time earlier. Joanne, the head nurse, quickly took over compressions from me and I was able to pull the stretcher out of the way. But there was too much activity for me to clear the stretcher out of the room. Bill was helping with the code, so I just stood there. However, while leaning back against the wall, the previous 36 hours caught up to me. I closed my eyes and despite the hectic noise of the code going on in front of me, I fell asleep.

Yes, I fell asleep standing up in an ER during a code. It didn't matter that there was an unholy commotion going on around me. I couldn't hear the cardiac monitor, nor the incessant squeak of the stretcher as Joanne thumped on our victim's chest. I was lost in my own little dream world. The next thing I remember is hearing Joanne, the ER nurse doing chest compressions, exclaim "Oh my God," and I woke up. Everyone was staring at me: the whole code had frozen as they turned to see me asleep against the wall. Holly, who was doing an ER rotation at the time, grabbed my arm and led me, dazed and confused, out of the room. I hadn't even noticed that Holly had been working the code with us until she tried to rescue me.

But the damage was done. I would forever be known as the person who fell asleep during a code. I got no sympathy from the rest of the ER or ambulance staff, despite the fact that I had been working for 36 hours straight. For the next few weeks, anytime there was a code, people would ask me if I needed a nap. Or if someone saw me yawning, they would promise me a code so I could get some extra sleep. So much for caring professionals. Except for Holly. She seemed to take pity on me and said she would check in every so often to make sure that I wasn't doing too many 36-hour shifts.

When I got back from the city and that marathon weekend, I realized that I had a chemistry exam the next morning. So I was facing a few more hours without sleep. I grabbed my stash of caffeine (instant coffee, instant hot chocolate and cola). I combined the coffee and hot chocolate for a kind of café mocha. The cola was for a cold jolt, while the coffee-chocolate was the hot. I went to the chemistry labs to study because the dorms were still very active and not conducive to studying.

The chemistry department was in a four-story brick building that dated to the late 1800s. It was very solid, with all the quirks and charm of an ancient edifice. Because it had been used as a science and biology building for so many years it had some unusual aspects—for example, there was a room that was lined with inch-thick lead, because it had been used to store radioactive chemicals. The chemistry building also used to have a major entomology program. Entomology is the study of bugs and there was once a huge insect colony on the premises, including exotic cockroaches. The official colony was long gone, but the building still housed a bizarre microenvironment of ants and cockroaches living and thriving in it. There were red ants, big black carpenter ants, fire ants, and black and red ants, and they all seemed more active at night.

The most interesting insects in the building were the cockroaches. They were huge and aggressive—often two or three inches long. You could actually hear the cockroaches scurrying across the tile floor, which made for an eerie late-night work environment. I could hear them scurrying away when I turned on the lights and sneaking around as I settled in to study.

I ignored all this and began studying my chemistry diligently. More than two days without sleep made it easy to filter out the noise and focus on the pages in front of me, and the caffeine helped keep me awake. I was learning physical chemistry and one topic I related to was entropy: the disorder and randomness in the universe. There was a lot of disorder and randomness on the ambulance and in the city, too. The city, like the universe, always tended towards greater disorder, increased entropy, with random violence from accidents and crime.

While I was memorizing the formulas I would need the next morning, I started to recognize the signs of extreme fatigue. I continued anyway, and at about 3 a.m. I felt a strange trembling in my left leg. I knew that muscle tremors and twitching could be a sign of excessive caffeine. I knew these tremors could also affect heart rhythm, so I took my pulse, which was normal. Nonetheless, I decided to go back to my room and some well-deserved sleep.

On the walk back to my dorm I wondered if I had pushed myself too far. I thought I knew how to handle caffeine, but could I have overdosed on it? Overdosing is something a drug addict does, not me. I took my pulse again and monitored my breathing. These were still normal. What was happening to me? I continued to my room worrying that I had become a caffeine addict. Nonetheless, sleep arrived quickly and it was deep and rewarding.

The next morning, when I woke to the clock radio as usual, news said that the area had been hit by a small earthquake at about 3 a.m. I immediately realized that my leg was trembling last night because it was leaning against the wall, and the wall had the tremor, not me. I was so relieved that I happily walked to the physical chemistry test that I was far from fully prepared for. I was never so happy to do so poorly in a test.

During my next shift I told Holly about my experience. At first she seemed concerned and even miffed at my apparent overdose—that is, until I got to the earthquake punch line. She said that I really needed someone to look after me when I was working in the big, bad college. She seemed to sympathize with the lack of sleep and was even concerned that I did poorly on the test.

"Hey, I still passed." I said.

"I bet you would ace those classes if you focused on them. Why do you pull so many shifts on the ambulance?"

"Do you have any suggestions as to how else I might be spending my time?" There was a long silence before I went on. "Why don't we go to a movie next Friday?"

"OK, it's a date!"

Vomit on the Ceiling

Why do they say things come in threes? One Saturday dayshift I learned why.

I hadn't worked the night before because Holly and I went to the movies. A first date to the movies is generally an easy one, because once the movie starts you don't have to worry about talking. Afterwards you can talk about whether you liked the movie or not. We wanted a non-violent, non-medical, non-sob-story, non-life-and-death movie, and there seems to be no such thing anymore, so we went to *The Rocky Horror Picture Show*. Holly had never been to one and I was an addict. I told her it was more than a movie; it was a movie plus a live show and also included songs like "The Time Warp" and "Sweet Transvestite." She was somewhat shocked by it all, but not disappointed. She especially liked the part about the lead character, Dr. Frank-N-Furter, doing biochemical research.

"Is that what you do in your lab?" she whispered to me.

"Yes, except for the dress." We had a good time, but went our separate ways after the movie. I had to be ready for a 7 a.m. shift the next morning.

Every emergency services person is eventually asked if he or she has ever seen or experienced anything which made them "lose it," usually meaning faint or vomit. That question has been put to me many times, and the shift this Saturday took me there, right to the edge of what I could take. I didn't lose it but I was very, very close.

That day I was working with Rick, an experienced paramedic who had worked as an army medic in Vietnam and often compared the maliciousness and animosity that the locals felt against the police, ambulance and fire personnel here to villagers he encountered in the jungles. His biggest complaint was that the ambulance personnel went to some of the most dangerous places in the city, often during or after violence, completely unarmed, while the locals had plenty of guns and other weapons. Rick, however, always carried a revolver on his ankle. I always felt safe when working with him.

Rick worked with one partner almost exclusively, but his partner was on vacation that week. Rick had a list of approved replacements, and I felt honored to be on it. Because I was considered a part-time employee, I didn't get to work with a regular partner. So I was pleased to have been scheduled with Rick for much of the week—working with the same partner gave you a chance to adjust to the rhythm of each other's behavior on the calls.

The day started harmlessly enough with our first call at 7:03 a.m. It came in as "man having a heart attack." Rick and I speeded to an exclusive and obscure back-street. The house was a beautiful single-family brown-stone that must have been more than 120 years old. Up on the second story, face down on the pristine white tiles of the bathroom floor was an elderly man with his pajamas around his ankles and diarrhea pooling between his legs. There was a strong smell of feces in the room, and we could tell that our patient was in full cardiac arrest.

Rick secured an airway to maintain the patient's breathing and I had to kneel in the warm, runny diar-rhea, slithering along the cold white tile while doing chest compressions. I didn't hesitate to let Rick drive afterward, because he was an excellent driver though a fast and aggressive one. In the back of the ambulance, I had to time ventilating (giving breaths of oxygen) between the screeching starts and stops as he muscled his way along the city streets to the hospital. The ambulance had a very good oxygen delivery system—excellent pressure that would inflate lungs at the push of a button. However, it did require that I keep the mask and tubing attached to my patient. Not an easy task in a fast-moving ambulance.

"Joe!" Rick screamed from the front.

"What?"

"Do you know what inertia is?"

I couldn't believe he was asking me a science question at a time like this.

Rick continued, "It's a new diarrhea medication that keeps you going and going and going. It seems our patient took too much of the stuff."

"Nice joke, Rick. Thanks."

I guess our patient was a little carsick (if that is possible with a patient in cardiac arrest) because during Rick's little joke, he vomited between ventilations. I saw this, of course, but the next acceleration by the speed demon made me fall on the vent and force high pressure oxygen into our patient and also send fresh vomit splattering over me, from my eyeglasses all the way down my face and chest. I was able to confirm that our patient had orange juice and oatmeal for breakfast—a great mix to have splashed in your face.

About now my breakfast was trying to make a return, too. The smell and taste of acidic, partially digested orange juice and fermenting oatmeal filled my senses and it took a tremendous amount of will power to suppress the contractions of my stomach, stifle a strong gag reflex and hold on as Rick screeched to another stop, all the while supplying O_2 to our patient. It was truly a Herculean effort to give my patient the medical care he deserved, but I did it despite the strong likelihood that he wouldn't make it out of the ER alive.

It was a tremendous relief when Rick opened the back door of the ambulance and let in fresh air. It didn't help much, however, when he immediately started to gag and loudly exclaim, "Oh my God, shit and vomit form a whole new smell experience."

Even though our patient's heart was beating when we brought him into the hospital (it had started and stopped several times during the call), he died that morning. But the smell on me and in the back of the ambulance lasted for the rest of the day. I desperately needed to change my shirt and pants. Fortunately, I always brought a spare shirt to work. Unfortunately, I didn't have a spare pair of uniform pants. The spare pants I did have were for a date with Holly. So soap and warm water was the best I could do. Even after washing my pants while wearing them, they retained a lingering odor of diarrhea. And there were 10 hours of shift to go.

The next call was right in front of the DMZ. The police station had a wide, flat parking lot, which led right to the main street. Kids loved to skateboard all through that area and when they fell and broke something, we got called.

When a 12-year-old boy's head meets a 40-year-old piece of concrete, the head loses every time. We arrived to find this boy lying next to his skateboard, unconscious and bleeding heavily from the head and nose. Rick and I worked together like a well-oiled machine and gave only passing notice to the police department supervisors watching from the DMZ. We were on show for the police and the neighborhood and doing a top-notch job was the best form of showing off. The boy, Stephen, was too big for our pediatrics equipment, so we put him on our adult backboard and immobilization equipment. Even though it dwarfed his small body, we secured him to the board like a mummy in its bandages.

Stephen was unconscious and we treated his injuries as very serious, but he was breathing on his own, so we didn't need the ventilation equipment. I had to keep a very close eye on Stephen as Rick made a slow and cautious trip to the ER, quite a contrast to the fast and furious ride with our dying diarrhea man. Because Stephen might have a head or spinal injury, Rick kept the stops and starts very smooth so as to avoid aggravating any injury. A three-minute ambulance ride became a 10-minute ride.

After the earlier mishap with the ventilator, slow was OK with me. OK that is until Stephen experienced a phenomenon called projectile vomiting. Stomach muscles are among the strongest in the body. Vomiting is the stomach and abdomen expelling the contents of the stomach, up the esophagus and out the mouth. For the body to vomit, the intestinal muscles must contract so that nothing goes into the intestine. At the same time, the muscles in the throat and esophagus relax. The stomach then quickly contracts and the laws of physics dictate that the contents exit the mouth. If the stomach contracts with enough force and speed, the stomach contents come out very fast and can travel a great distance. The result is projectile vomit.

With no warning, our passenger had the most voluminous projectile vomit I ever saw. The vomit came out so forcefully that it hit the ceiling of the ambulance. I quickly determined that Stephen had recently eaten a large amount of cookies and chocolate milk. This pasty mixture was now plastered on the ceiling of the ambulance. There was no time for me to marvel at the splatter pattern, though—I had to secure Stephen's airway. The risk now was that he would aspirate the vomit into his lungs and cause damage that could lead to pneumonia. I rolled the backboard and Stephen towards me and cleared his mouth of vomit. Stephen was so well secured to the backboard that he didn't shift position when I rolled him on his side. I needed to lean over Stephen while holding him on his side and prevent him from drawing any of the vomit into his lungs. As I did this the vomit on the ceiling dripped down onto me. I could feel it slithering down my back and drying in my hair. But, there was nothing I could do, because I couldn't let go of Stephen. I had to endure the rest of that long, slow ambulance ride in this position with no escape from the rain of vomit.

When Rick opened the back door of the ambulance, he asked a simple question. "Why am I not surprised by this smell?"

Stephen turned out to be fine. They told us later that the first thing he said when he woke up was, "Where's my skateboard?"

Now I needed to change shirts again. I ended up putting the first vomit-spattered shirt back on, because it was the lesser of two evils. So I was ready for the next call with shit on my knees and vomit on my chest (as well as on my back and hair). All this had happened before noon and, boy, was I looking forward to lunch—these things in no way affected my appetite.

Stephen had been skateboarding to enjoy the warm and dry Saturday and our next call was the result of a guy out taking advantage of the good weather by breaking in a new motorcycle. Everyone knows the only way to break in a new motorcycle is to take it out on the open road and see how fast it can go. On his brand new bike, Art had easily passed 100 mph on a long straightaway of a four-lane road. The road conditions were great, and Art had both lanes clear. Clear, that is, until a tow truck decided to make a U-turn in front of speeding Art. The result was that Art and his bike hit the side of the truck with tremendous force.

Art's body hit the boom of the tow truck so hard that the boom was bent, and you could literally say that he had made an impression. His arms and body were severely deformed by the impact. Two ambulances were sent to this accident because of its severity, so we had four people working furiously to give Art every chance to make it. We had two IVs in his mangled arms to give him fluids because he had lost a lot of blood. There were also more pressing things to worry about, like the organ damage inside his chest and abdomen.

I was doing compressions on Art's chest and could feel the broken ribs grinding together with each compression. There was blood everywhere and my hands and arms were covered in clotting and drying blood. The scene was a mess.

Traffic was backed up because the accident took up two lanes of the four-lane highway. Cars were passing slowly and often stopped to watch. I hate rubberneckers. They have no consideration for others—not the emergency personnel, the victim, nor their fellow travelers. All they do is gawk. I was facing traffic and I got to see the shocked expressions of the rubberneckers as they passed. One guy in a shiny new convertible Mercedes had stopped and was forcefully gesturing for his female passenger to have a look. She was a stunningly attractive blonde wearing Ray-Ban sunglasses, shaking her head in refusal. He kept up the prompting and she eventually did turn towards this horrific scene. I could see her eyes open wide through the dark tint of her sunglasses. A life in tatters and near death, on the ground, blood streaming from the mangled body, is a sight no one should be forced to see. After taking this in, she slowly and calmly turned toward the front of the car, leaned forward and started to vomit. As she did so, her Ray-Bans slid off her face and dangled in front of her, held in place by an eyeglass retainer. Her next retch produced a flood that hit her glasses and bounced off in all directions. The guy driving the Mercedes had an expression of shock as vomit splattered all over his car and I felt that he deserved the mess spewing from his girlfriend's mouth. It seemed like justice being served to rubberneckers and to this guy in particular. I did feel sorry for the poor woman, but I started to laugh.

Remember, the scene is a true horror with probably mortal injuries, and I suddenly I start to laugh. No one else had seen the vomiting blonde, so my laughter seemed very out of place. Inappropriate laughter can be a sign of burnout or even mental illness. There is a lot of gallows humor and sick jokes in emergency work, but laughing for no apparent reason or in the midst of a tragedy can be a bad sign. Rick, obviously concerned, stopped what he was doing and with great sincerity asked if I was OK. All I could say was that I was fine. I promised to explain later and silently said to myself that I was relieved it wasn't me who got vomited on this time. Things do seem to come in threes, and this was vomit number three for me today.

Ambulance people do usually try to follow up on their patients by reading the papers regularly, the obituaries especially. The obituaries are often the final chapter, revealing at least a fraction of the impact our ambulance call had. The list of grieving family members gives us some idea of the many people who are feeling the loss. We often heard about the bad outcomes and only rarely about the happy endings. For us, a good outcome would be a patient who left the ambulance and emergency room alive. Sometimes a transport ambulance crew would notice that they were bringing home a victim of a previous call and would take the time to tell us how they were doing. Going home was usually a happy ending.

Later, Rick and I were in the ER dropping off an elderly woman from a nursing home. After transferring the patient, Holly told me she had a surprise for me in the quiet room. I eagerly followed her there and was surprised to find a half-eaten cake that was shaped and frosted to look like a full-size skateboard. Holly told me that Stephen's family had come in and dropped it off for "the people who helped Stephen." I was glad someone seemed to think that the system was working. Maybe I really was "helping people." Holly and I shared a happy moment in the quiet room as we enjoyed the cake together.

Angel Dust

Angel dust—or PCP, or phencyclidine, or whatever you want to call it—is a hallucinogenic drug that causes people to "dissociate." Their minds and bodies seem to separate and they have no perception of pain or memory of the events during a trip. Calling this type of drug episode a "trip" is a perfect description, because they left their bodies, left reality and went elsewhere. I don't pretend to understand the psychology or chemistry of what happens to these people, but I do know they are dangerous. Not only have they lost all sense of reality and understanding of right and wrong, but if they get pissed off, they have the strength to take revenge on whomever they think has wronged them. I've seen people who were "dusted" rip down doors and bend cast iron. They are able to do these things because they do not feel the pain which would normally be telling them to stop. So, when they are pounding on a door, they can hit harder and harder, until the door is kindling and no longer a barrier. Their arm may be hurting too, but they aren't aware of it and they don't care.

Angel dust is scary. A dusted person may not know he is injured. But what is worse is that he may decide that the ambulance crew or police are the bad guys and may attack us. If that happens, there is only one thing to do: "beat feet," run, bug out, abandon ship. When the dust trip ends, the brain and body will start to talk to each other again and the patient will seek help, often not remembering what happened or how they got injured.

There were growing concerns in EMS circles about ambulances catching fire. The putative cause was that many of the ambulances were retrofitted with a second gas tank. During the retrofit, the gas line was run near the exhaust system. If the exhaust system got too hot, the thinking was that it might ignite the gas in the fuel line. Several ambulances had recently caught fire, and the second fuel line was suspected as the culprit. We tried to make a habit of not leaving the vehicle idling for long periods, especially on hot days, but one of our ambulances did catch fire—fortunately, when I was not working. No one was injured and the patient was transported by another crew. There was the usual finger-pointing and teeth-gnashing after the fire, but no one got in trouble. We were short an ambulance for a few weeks before the replacement finally arrived, and it was a beautiful thing. I am not sure how the fuel line problem was fixed, but fires eventually stopped happening.

One hazy, hot and humid summer evening, several police cars and the ambulance were dispatched to a "domestic dispute with shots fired." We did not get a chance to treat any GSWs because when we arrived we were greeted by more shots being fired—at us. This was a new experience for me. Our next surprise was the flames coming from the windows of the house. The cops all had their guns in one hand and radios in the other. Every one of the police officers at the scene was calling for backup and the fire department. We got the ambulance out of there to avoid being blocked in by the FD. When the FD arrived to fight the fire, they too were treated to the experience of being shot at. One firefighter turned to my partner Bill Smith and exclaimed, "I just got fucking shot at!" Bill, always the comic, responded with his best Curly imitation: "And they only predicted rain."

By now the police had the house surrounded. We thought some people had been shot or injured inside the house, but we couldn't help them. The fire department wouldn't fight the fire because they didn't want to be shot. The police couldn't make contact with anyone in the house, so we just waited. Eventually, Bill and I were dispatched to another call—this one with visibly injured people and no one shooting at us.

Bill and I didn't get back to that scene until our next shift together, the next day, when the medical examiner (ME) was there to recover the bodies from the burnt ruins. As the story went, some guy had been tripping on dust at a party when he announced he was going to go kill his ex-wife. He succeeded in doing as he had announced, along with killing his ex-mother-in-law. The ME had verified two charred female bodies in the rubble. But no gun or male body had been found so far. There was a lot of debris to search yet, so the case was not closed. Bill and I would have to follow up on this call later to see if the body count changed.

Elsewhere in the city, the PD detectives were continuing the investigation of this killing by interviewing friends, colleagues and neighbors. People offered the usual platitudes ("It's such a tragedy," "We never expected this to happen here"), but there was one curious twist to the story. When the detectives went to get a statement from the former employer of the dusted shooter, they started in the usual way by saying, "Are you the employer of Mr. X?" The response was, "Yeah, he's in back." Obviously, the detectives were surprised to hear that a presumed crispy critter was working today, so they went to investigate. What they found out became a legend in the department. Our dusted shooter woke up in some alley that morning and went to work. He had no recollection of the previous evening's events. He still had the gun in his pocket, with no bullets left. A surprise for him, but not for the detectives, because he had emptied his revolver the night before into his ex-wife and her mother.

Angel dust is no fun.

I think there might have been a bad batch of the stuff in the city that summer, because Bill and I got another dusted patient that evening. A radio dispatcher said that a cop car was "in pursuit" and gave a street address and direction of pursuit. We waited for an update but heard nothing. We wanted to know where the chase was headed, because a lot of these high-speed pursuits end in an accident that would require an ambulance.

We finally got the information we needed in a message that said "ambulance needed at scene." So off we went, not knowing what had happened, but confident in our assumption that there had been an MVA.

What had happened was this: a police officer in a cruiser had started to chase a car for driving suspiciously—as in driving on the sidewalk and running over parking meters. Fortunately, no one on the street was injured. At the end of the street, the car went straight into a brick building, which was also unhurt. The driver was uninjured too, though his car was heavily damaged. The PO approached the car, gun drawn, to see a solitary ARP inhaling and swallowing dust.

"What are you doing?" the cop asked.

The ARP stopped, looked up, and said, "Cleaning up."

This was a dangerous response, because it meant he had just "cleaned up" a large amount of dust by taking it into his body. With gun holstered and two other officers on scene as backup, the PO started cuffing the dusted gang member. But when the first cuff was on, the ARP decided the cop was a bad guy and punched him in the jaw. The ARP had superhuman strength by now, so it took three PO's to cuff one of his hands to an iron railing. But he still had one hand free, which was flailing at the three officers.

I did not need to be told the rest of the conversation between the POs there. It went like this:

"Cop-shop?"

"Nope, ER."

Translation: "Do you want to take him to the police station?"

"No, too much paperwork. Let the ambulance and hospital ER deal with him until the dust wears off."

Anyway, when we arrived at the scene there were four POs in a semicircle around this ARP who was cuffed to the railing. The guy was wildly swinging at the cops just out of his reach. They were leaning in towards the ARP and taunting him to swing at them; he would strike out in their direction and they would lean back and let the arm swoosh harmlessly past them. Bill and I brought a Reeves stretcher, which consisted of long, thin strips of wood slid into cloth slots, so it could be rolled up like a paper scroll. It was ideal for restraining dangerous patients, because once you got it on them they were cocooned in it. Bill and I got soft and set up the Reeves stretcher on the ground just out of reach of the ARP. We were holding a set of triangular bandages and rolling them into ropelike restraints, which we would use to tie the patient's hands and feet.

Bill and I positioned ourselves to the right and left of the ARP, looking for a chance to take him down. Our chance arrived when he seemed to suddenly understand the situation—he stood straight up and asked in a surprisingly clear and coherent voice, "What are you guys doing?" At that moment, Bill tackled him high, I went low, and we scissored him to the ground. Bill secured the ARP's free arm and I got his legs with the help of Pete the cop, who unlocked the gang member from the railing). Pete was the one who'd been hit in the mouth earlier and I noticed his lips were getting fuller from the swelling. The three of us put the ARP face down on the stretcher, with both hands tied behind his back and feet tied together. He was now wrapped like a sausage. "That's the fastest immobilization I've ever seen," one of the other cops said.

"Joe and I have similar tastes in women," Bill shot back. This comment strengthened my suspicion that Bill might be one of those helping ambulance and ER restraints to go missing.

Pete accompanied us to the ER because his supervisor said he needed to have his swollen lip looked at. Pete and I were in the back of the rig with the ARP for the ride. En route, the ARP started to wriggle like a worm and actually started to squeeze forward through the front of the Reeves stretcher. To stop him from making an escape, I employed an old-fashioned restraining technique: I sat on him. This made our dusted ARP even madder. As he tried even harder to squeeze out of the stretcher, he also told me, in Spanish, things I should do to my mother. I was not a big believer in Freud's views on Oedipus, so I simply told him to shut up, in both Spanish and English. Pete was happy to help with the restraining of the ARP, and he sat next to me on the guy's chest. The combined weight of the two of us assured a safe ride to the hospital. Being a conscientious health care provider, I got up to let him breathe every minute or two.

When we arrived in the ER, they had a room prepared and two security guards plus an orderly ready to help. We got the ARP transferred to a hospital gurney and restrained him with brand new, fresh-from-the-box leather restraints with lamb's wool liners and no blood-stains on them. Bill eyed these enviously as we tied down all four points: that is, his arms and legs were tied to the four corners of the gurney, to a background of curses and screams.

Because Bill had knotted the ambulance restraints too tightly, we were forced to cut them off the ARP's wrists, and I had to use heavy-duty scissors to do this. This little job was complicated by the fact that the hos-pital restraints were in the way. As I cut through our restraints the ARP (who was in no way harmed by this) started screaming at me to stop and yelled, "What are you doing?"

Before I could respond, Pete the cop answered, "He's cutting off your hand so you can't punch any more cops." In a somewhat lucid voice, the ARP asked me if this were true. Without hesitating I said, "What do you think?" I showed him the heavy-duty surgical scissors, entirely free of blood, and went back to cutting the remnants of the restraints. Nonetheless, he screamed again. I ignored it as Pete cheered, "Cut the bone, cut the bone!" I tried to admonish Pete to let me finish, because the ARP's squirming made it difficult to cut through the restraints. But I also knew the torment was good therapy for him, so I was half-hearted in my pro-tests. The two security guards watched in amusement the guy who was convinced his arm was being amputated. I made a feeble attempt to keep Pete quiet, but did nothing more to convince the ARP otherwise.

Eventually the noise from our cubicle attracted attention. The head ER nurse, Joan, came storming in like a schoolmarm demanding, "What's going on here?"

Pete and I were caught like two naughty schoolboys, and I immediately confessed. "He thinks I'm cutting off his hand so he can't punch any more cops." The security guards, Pete and I stood there with heads bowed, fully expecting some sort of reprimand, because we permitted the ARP to think that and tormented him in that way.

Joan was shocked, but she also knew the ARP could feel no pain and would have no recollection of these events. Moreover, she understood Pete's need to gain some kind of closure from this incident. So she was understanding and forgiving—she turned to the ARP and said, "I wouldn't blame them if they did. Now keep quiet!" Then she walked out without looking at us, closing the door behind her. I went back to cutting and the ARP back to yelling.

About 10 minutes later, Pete, Bill and I were reminiscing in the ED about the call, when my favorite nursing student came to us and reported that she found Joan laughing in her office. When Holly asked Joan why she was laughing alone in her office she replied, "Ask the ambulance guys." So, Holly wanted to know what we did to make the sternest nurse in the hospital laugh hysterically, and I replied, "Gave a guy quality care."

"Remind me to never be injured around you guys," said Holly.

The disappearance of restraints from the ED was becoming problematic because the replacements often went missing and we were left with the old pair that was weakening, falling apart, covered with stains, and had blood, vomit, feces and who knows what else imbedded in the material. Multiple replacements had been purchased and quickly disappeared.

Nurse Rothchild (we called her Nurse Ratched) came up with a solution. She obtained a new set of restraints and had them delivered to her office. At the end of one busy night shift, she brought out the new pair for the beginning of the following shift. She had "pre-pared" the restraints the night before, however, by adding food coloring stains of red, brown and green. She announced to the new shift that these brand new restraints had been ruined by the previous shift and held up the colorfully marked pair to prove it. The stains were a great ruse. She reinforced the story with complaints about the constant theft of restraints, discouraging any further purchase of new and clean ones.

The result was an extended period with no loss of restraints, thanks to Nurse Ratched's little strategy. Unfortunately, one day a senior administrator came down to the ED for some kind of inspection tour and found the restraints to be "disgusting and unsanitary." They were replaced immediately and the old ones thrown away. When the new restraints arrived, of course, they quickly disappeared.

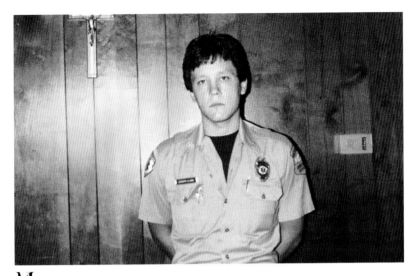

My first day of work as a professional EMT, at age 18.

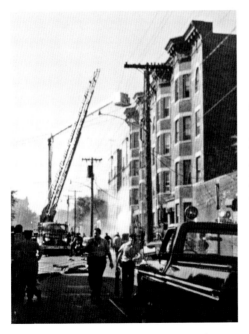

The Fire Department finishes fighting an apartment blaze as my EMT colleagues wrap up their work.

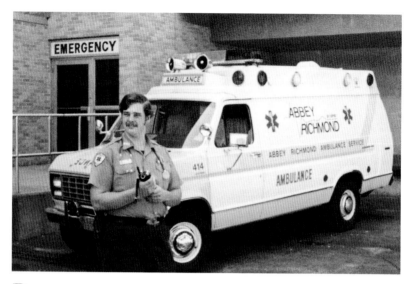

Bob Smith in front of an ambulance soon after starting on the job.

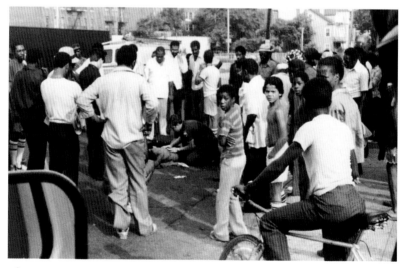

A colleague checks the condition of a cyclist hit by a truck.

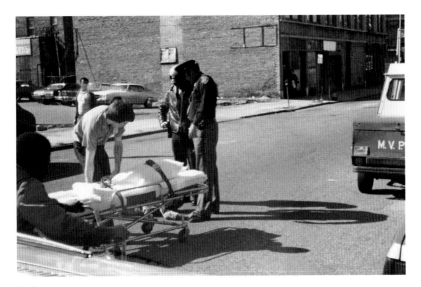

Here, an intoxiated man is lying on the ground holding a police officer's foot as EMT prepares the stretcher.

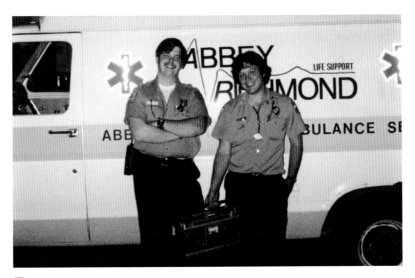

Bob Smith and I start a shift, complete with a forbidden boom box.

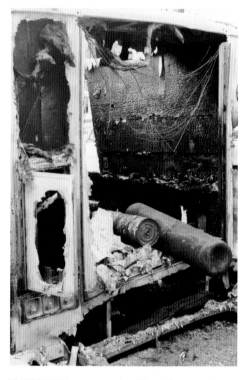

The ruined interior and exterior of an ambulance I sometimes drove which caught fire after retrofitting. Luckily, no one was injured.

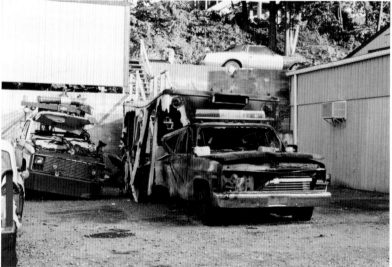

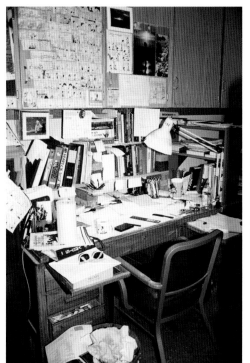

This is my desk at college. I had two lives, one on the ambulance, one at college, and tried to balance the two.

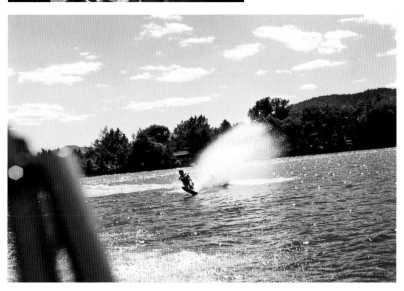

Shortly after this picture was taken, I hit a motor boat and ended up being taken to hospital in an ambulance.

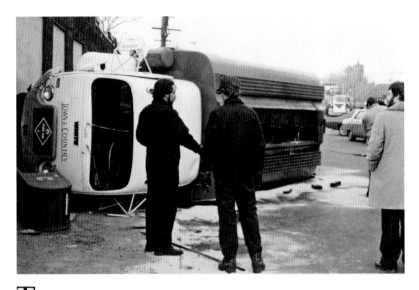

This oil tanker rollover had a good outcome, unlike some of the truck rollover calls we had.

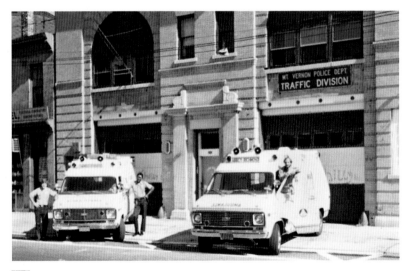

The garage door on the left crashed down on my ambulance a short time later.

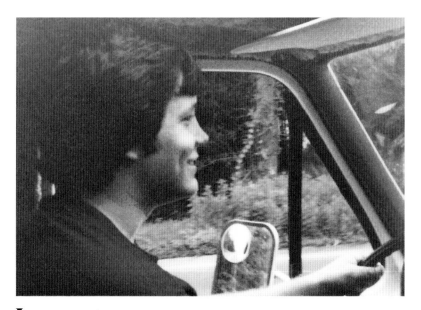

I always looked more relaxed on one of my rare days off.

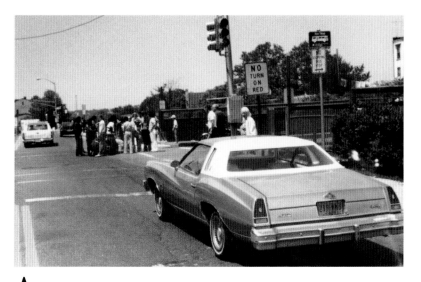

A crowd has already gathered around a man suffering from a seizure as we pull up to help.

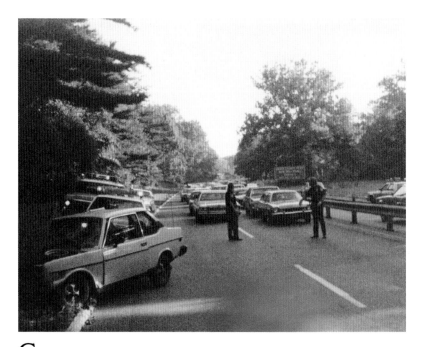

County Police held up traffic during morning rush hour so we could reach the scene of a crash.

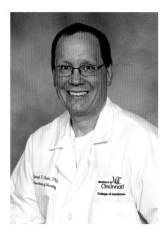

Today I am studying the causes and treatment of stroke at the University of Cincinnati

The Streets

When working on the ambulance, you become a part of the streets because you are always working in them. I could tell the time of day by the volume and direction of the traffic flow on certain commuter streets. Most people associate a street with a friend or colleague who lives there. Not me. I might forget the name of a street, but I would always remember the devastating car accident that happened there.

You might think it would be fun to drive an ambulance with lights and sirens, but it's not. There are lots of things to watch out for, such as the possibility that the car in front of you would pull into your lane. Sometimes drivers would do the craziest and most dangerous things when they saw an ambulance in their rear-view mirror. For example, I was driving with lights and sirens to a call of "man down" when I noticed a Corvette in front of me accelerate. This generally meant the person wanted to quickly get to a place to pull over. We were traveling along one of the parkways in the fast lane and most of the traffic was immediately pulling into the slow lane to let us pass. This Corvette did not move to the right. There were plenty of gaps in the traffic to pull over, so I was confused. I hit the siren and changed its tones to get the driver's attention, but still the car would not get out of my way. There was a long space in the right lane beside us, so I did something I normally wouldn't do: I tried to pass on the right. But the Corvette accelerated and would not let me pass. The driver even edged to the right to block me.

This was a tricky situation, so I ended up slowing down and opening a very safe distance from the Vette and continued on. Suddenly, there was a whoosh on the right: a police car had passed me and signaled the Vette to pull over. To my surprise, the driver did pull over and we passed both vehicles.

The police officer then radioed us and asked us to return to that location on the parkway when our call was done. I advised him that we would be a while because we were just en route to the call and he responded with, "I will be here with this driver until you get back to fill out the complaint." From the tone of his voice, I could tell the PO was furious.

We went back to the parkway after the call and our PO rescuer was still there with the red Corvette. He briefed us on what the driver had said. She denied preventing us from passing her on the right or left and insisted that her car could go much faster than a big old ambulance if she had wanted to. Therefore, it should have been obvious to us that she could not be blocking us.

It turned out that she had received three speeding tickets since purchasing the car and thought we would run interference against the police radar. As long as she kept in front of us, she figured she wouldn't get a speeding ticket. Her logic was lost on us and the PO. Her attempt to avoid getting a fourth speeding ticket was also unsuccessful. Moreover, she was given a citation for reckless driving and obstructing emergency personnel.

Another stupid but common thing that people do is follow a speeding ambulance. This is extremely risky because as soon as the ambulance passes, the cars we passed usually pull back into traffic. A small car with no lights or sirens is easy to hit. Normally, these drivers don't go so far as to run red lights when following an ambulance. I wish I could say that this never happened, but it did.

We were having trouble with our handheld police radio one day, so the dispatcher called us to police headquarters to get a new one. You got into dispatch area through the back door of the HQ. You had to go down the stairs to the basement, where the main dispatch was tucked away, surrounded by tons of equipment, including powerful computers. The room was (at least theoretically) bomb- and fireproof so it could store the tapes and records required to keep the police department in communication with the rest of the world in the event of a disaster. I had been there several times and had become friends with one of the senior dispatchers, Richie. Richie had wanted to be a regular patrol officer but was unable to work the streets because of a chronic back problem. He was a wannabe and ran the dispatch office like his own little fiefdom. When things got serious in the streets, Richie could make life for the PD very difficult or very easy. Richie would barter a light shift for a crew in exchange for a favor. For example, Bill Smith set Richie up on a blind date with the woman Richie eventually married. It was rumored that for two weeks after that date, Richie only sent Bill on the best calls.

Despite all the high-tech equipment, dispatch constantly had problems with the video surveillance system at the back entrance. There was no key to this door; because dispatch was open 24 hours a day, 7 days a week, access was only through confirmation of a recognized or expected person in the surveillance monitor. But when it was not working—which was most of the time—you had to use the intercom. This required a password and Richie had come up with the perfect one. We went up to the door, rang the buzzer and waited. When a crackling voice came over the speaker asking, "Who is it?" the necessary response was, "I'm a fucking terrorist," which I gladly said and we were let in.

While we were there, Bill and I were sent on a call, so we grabbed a new radio and left. The call was to the home of an elderly woman who was having chest pain. When we arrived, her husband met us dressed in a tweed jacket with a matching hat. During the call, he doted on his wife and tried to direct what we were doing. For the woman's heart attack, we did all the usual things to monitor her and get her relatively stabilized. I told her husband which hospital we were taking her to and reminded him to bring her ID, some personal effects such as a toothbrush and overnight bag and to lock the door when he left. Spouses and other loved ones were often anxious and absent-minded during emergencies, so it helped to gently remind them of these simple things. Occasionally, we would arrange for the police to give them a ride, but he seemed calm and intelligent, so we didn't push it when he said he wanted to drive himself to the hospital. I told him where to park and how to make his way to the ER. He assured me that he understood and would meet us at the hospital shortly.

While I was driving to the hospital with lights and sirens, I noticed a car tailgating us and speeding through the lights behind us. Because this was so dangerous, I kept an eye on the car behind me as well as the traffic in front as I made my way through the busy city traffic. Our shadow continued through the rest of the lights with us, including the red lights. It suddenly occurred to me to ask the woman we were transporting who was in no obvious distress what kind of car her husband drove. "A black BMW," she responded. An exact description of the car behind us.

I told Bill that I had to stop the ambulance for a second. Because our patient was quite stable, he consented, and I turned off the siren and pulled over, leaving the lights on. The BMW pulled over right behind us. I got out of the ambulance and ran to the car just as our patient's husband was getting out. "Is she OK? What's the problem?"

"She's fine. You, sir, are the problem. I want you to stay here for one full minute and make your own way to the hospital. Following us through the red lights like that is very dangerous."

"I hit the horn as I went through the lights," he said defensively.

"There's no discussion here. If you continue, I'll pull over again and wait until the police come. And they *will* make you wait. I won't be responsible for your accident. Do not move as we pull away." I stormed off.

He didn't follow immediately behind us this time, but he did arrive at the ER even before we had his wife out of the back of the ambulance. Bill came to me later, after the paperwork was done, and informed me that the husband had approached him. I immediately thought that the man was going to complain about my behavior, but instead Bill told me the man had given us each a $20 tip. I really didn't want to take the money. Bill said that the husband had anticipated that I would refuse, so he gave it to Bill and scurried off. I didn't want to confront the BMW driver again, so that tip paid for 10 minutes of one of my organic chemistry classes. I would have preferred an apology and no argument in the street. The street was my domain and I was not going to have this well intentioned guy make it more dangerous than it already was.

The next day I was working with Jay Lewis, and we had to go back to HQ and park the ambulance in the garage to restock our equipment. The ambulance garage was about 110 years old; it even had a place to load horse feed and muck out the horseshit. The building definitely had character. After we loaded our supplies, we took the chance to have a break and decompress. The ambulance was parked facing out of the garage with the big doors rolled down in front of it. The garage doors were thick and heavy. They made a lot of noise as they rumbled up and down, but when closed, they cut down on a lot of the street noise, and we needed the quiet.

Our respite didn't last long, because we were soon called out again. Jay hopped in the driver's seat and I went over to press the button that raised the garage door. I watched the door roll up, then I gave Jay the thumbs-up and he pulled out. But to my surprise when the big heavy door hit the top of the garage, it immediately began to fall back down. I kept hitting the up button, but the motor had cut out and the garage door slid down again. Jay was only part of the way out when the door hit the roof of our ambulance and took off all the lights and sirens as the ambulance rolled forward.

Our ambulance was now naked, but it could still be used to aid patients, and we headed to the call. En route, I advised dispatch what had happened, requested a loaner ambulance (which we called "leased lightning") and a police escort to lead us to the hospital from the call. Then Jay and I limped to the call, picked up our patient and bought her to the ER.

Well, the entire EMS system had heard me describe what had happened on the radio and they were well prepared for us. They had several signs drawn on hospital sheets hanging over the ambulance bay when we arrived. One said, "Garage Door Open—Ambulance Can Pass." Another showed a big Band Aid with the caption, "Place on ambulance boo-boos." The last one said, "If you want service in the ER, please blow siren." (Because my surname is Clark and I was working with Jay Lewis on that shift, the whole escapade became known as "The Lewis and Clark expedition.")

Jay and I finished the shift in the leased lightning and struggled to get acquainted with the new rig. There is always an unsettling feeling about being in a strange ambulance; they all drive differently and have their own little quirks. We were still checking out our new wheels when we got a serious call downtown. "Pedestrian hit by car—and dragged" was the way the call came in and it had an ominous ring. I had never heard Richie use such a solemn emphasis.

I drove us to a crowded part of the city, an area with lots of pedestrians on the sidewalks and streets crammed with cars. We arrived to find a very messy scene. There was a cop standing over a well-built male dressed in an expensive gray business suit. The patient was on the ground with his left leg hooked by the back bumper of a cream-colored Lincoln Continental. The Lincoln's bumper was bent and pulled out, but it looked to me like the car's damage was old and not likely to have been caused by dragging this guy. The injuries to the victim were fatal: a large part of the back of his head had been scraped off as he was dragged two blocks behind the Lincoln. His scalp and hair trailed from the top of his head like thick, bloody dreadlocks. This scraping along the road formed a blood/brain skid mark that stretched the entire distance he was dragged. I guess if he was dragged farther nothing would have been left, but we could have followed the trail to the driver's home.

The woman who owned the Lincoln had indeed been driving with a damaged bumper when she made a right turn and cut the wheel too hard. This caused the car to jump up onto the crowded curb. This poor gentleman was standing at the curb, waiting to cross the street, when the ragged edges of the broken bumper hooked a large chunk of muscle on his lower leg, upended him and dragged him along the street. The driver thought the drag was due to hitting the curb, so she kept moving as people tried to flag her down. She ignored the pedestrians waving at her, she said, because she "had the right of way." When questioned by the police, she also said that the accident couldn't be her fault because she had told her husband to fix the car's bumper. This, she claimed, exonerated her from any responsibility. The victim, meanwhile, had nothing to say about it. We collected as much of his skull, brain, skin and hair as we could and brought him to the hospital—DOA.

Shake and Bake and Other Ambulance Regulars

The city was full of victims, whether of freak accidents or of circumstances. And then there were the professional victims—the people who constantly called the ambulance for trivial or imaginary complaints. This was an abuse of the service and it was supposed to be illegal. But very few people were ever charged with this crime—we simply had to deal with them whenever they called.

If I were to say that the city streets were my home, that would be a metaphor. But for these people, the streets really were their home. Many hardworking citizens with real jobs and nice homes tried to ignore them, pretending they did not see that guy urinating in the alley. But the ambulance would come for these people— sometimes repeatedly.

An interesting couple who lived in the streets was Sally and Vince DeMayr. DeMayr was not the man's real last name. I had no idea what his last name actually was, but he was prominent among the street people and he just started calling himself "the Mayor." So Vince the Mayor became Vince DeMayr. Vince was an alcoholic, and the booze took much of his money. But he did have a hobby: starting fires. Vince was a pyromaniac.

Sally supposedly had blonde hair, but she never washed it, so it always looked brown and greasy. Sally was not a substance abuser, or "subab" in our lingo; in fact, she did not like taking any kind of drugs. She felt that drugs were the way the government controlled people. Unfortunately, Sally *should* have taken drugs: that is, she was an epileptic who needed medications to control her profound seizures, which are called grand mal or tonic-clonic seizures. These would result in injuries to her arms, legs, head and face. The EMS people generally agreed that Sally knew when a seizure was coming on. She would then go from her hidden home to a public place and wait for the seizure to come. People would see poor Sally and call the ambulance—even the most hardened city resident seeing one of her seizures would call 911. For Sally, this was a windfall. She would be taken to the hospital, cleaned up, and given a warm meal and a clean bed to sleep in.

Well, Sally and Vince shared the same cardboard abode for a time and Sally got pregnant. She received little prenatal care because she didn't trust the authorities and didn't want to take any drugs. But she did avail herself of all the free food and clothing the welfare services gave her. I think that she was even housed for a while during her pregnancy. Sally and Vince were blessed with a baby boy and they named him Steven Benjamin and called him S.B.

The emergency services got to know little S.B. because he inherited both of his parents' traits. He was an epileptic like his mother and a pyromaniac like his father. We called him S.B. as well, but for us the initials stood for "Shake and Bake," his two most notable characteristics. S.B. tended to have a seizure when he got excited and the thing that got him most excited was setting fires. Therefore, it was easy to catch him: he would be in front of the fire having a seizure when the FD arrived. This gave people in the crowd the option of watching the fire or watching us on the ambulance treat young Mr. S.B. DeMayr.

Nick Bariglio was a classic subab. His life could be divided into four unequal parts: Part One was getting high, mainly from injecting heroin into his veins. Part Two was sleeping it off. Part Three was stealing money to score more drugs, and Part Four was condescending to take methadone when he could not get enough heroin. Nick never called it heroin; he thought heroin was "a female hero." He called it "stuff," and it gave him freedom from the real world, especially if he got "good stuff." We would occasionally pick Nick up when he was on a bad trip, but one day while tripping, Nick walked in front of a car and sustained serious head injuries. I tried to assess Nick's level of consciousness, but between the head injury and the drugs in his system, this was hard to judge. His injuries were severe and his life was in danger, but it turned out that Nick was lucky that day and he recovered, albeit with memory loss and profound brain damage. His personality was dulled, all his emotions were blunted and he could only walk with a slow shuffle. The injury simply accelerated what the drugs were doing.

When Nick was discharged from the hospital, he was no longer able to make a living by stealing. Because of his severe disability he became a ward of the state, unable to work. Nick was reduced to the regular methadone clinic, but still craved shooting up. A clever hospital intern—or "intard," as we called them—had a small brainstorm (we called it a brain drizzle). He wanted to find out if Nick was still capable of shooting up or if that skill had been lost in the accident. The intard provided a sterile syringe filled with a saltwater solution, which Nick quickly injected. With great relief and excitement, Nick proclaimed the salt solution to be "good stuff"; he could now get a rush from the act of shooting up and did not seem to need the drug to get high. Over time, a little arrangement was established in the hospital clinic whereby Nick was weaned off methadone and self-administered saltwater instead.

John Dossi was an experienced paramedic with the bedside manner of Florence Nightingale when he needed it, but a cynical and gritty sense of humor about the job. John was an avid sailor and his upper body was incredibly strong. With his slim build and powerful arms he looked like Popeye—all he needed were anchor tattoos on his forearms and a pipe. One day John and I were called to a project house. The call did not come from the house, because these people did not have a phone. Someone had run to a local store to ask them to dial 911. The call came in as "kid not breathing," so we pulled out all the stops to get there. John and I hustled up the stairs, but we slowed down for the last few flights, because we knew the baby was not in any danger: we could hear the baby crying as the mother screamed for us, and when a baby is crying, it must be breathing.

The tiny apartment was really the attic of this rundown boarding house and because it was August it was very hot. There was no phone, no air conditioning—very few comforts in this dim and dismal place. The mother, still clutching the crying baby, said that the little girl had stopped breathing while asleep. So she did what any mother would do: she screamed, grabbed the baby and ran frantically around the apartment. According to the mother, her love for the baby was what brought her back from the hands of death. The mother wouldn't give the baby to me, but I checked the girl out while Mom held on and found that the baby's chest was congested. I asked if the baby had had a cold and the mother said yes. John then asked to see where the baby slept. The four of us walked to a corner of the room where a blanket covered a makeshift bassinet. I felt the bed cushion and it was warm and moist with sweat from the baby. I asked if the baby had been laying flat on her back in the bassinet? Mom said yes.

John and I then explained that the baby had likely had fluid build-up in her lungs while lying flat in the hot, humid bassinet and this could stop her breathing for a period. We told the mother that the baby should be OK sleeping someplace less hot and humid. We said we could take them to the hospital and the welfare people would try to find a better place for the baby to sleep. So off we went.

John drove while I sat in back getting details from the mother, Ms. Jones. There was no Mr. Jones, and I took down necessary information from the mother. The drive to the hospital was taking a while because we were going without lights and sirens to allow the baby to sleep. The baby was breathing fine in the air conditioning of the ambulance, so I decided to make small talk.

"What's the baby's name?"

"Famalley," Ms. Jones replied. At least, that's what it sounded like.

"That's a pretty name. Where did it come from?"

"The hospital," was the simple reply.

"You decided to name her Famalley in the hospital?"

"No, the hospital gave her the name."

"What do you mean the hospital gave her the name?"

"The hospital named my baby," she said firmly.

How on earth could the hospital name the baby? I thought a while, and then asked, "Wait, how do you spell her name?"

"You know, F-E-M-A-L-E—Famalley."

And it hit me. This woman had gone to the hospital to have the baby. The newborn was given a little ID bracelet with "FEMALE Jones" written on it. The mother interpreted this as the hospital's name for the baby and simply accepted it. Social services were going to love this case. I couldn't wait to report to the nurses at the ED.

The summer heat continued over Labor Day weekend, and I was working 32 hours over that Friday, Saturday and Sunday. I would be going back to college soon, so I needed the money. The summer party season was coming to an end, and as Labor Day approached people wanted to take advantage of the nice weather before fall arrived. The ambulance was busy that weekend. John and I went to a derelict building known to be a drug house for an "unconscious woman" call.

Calls like this were always difficult and dangerous, because it was relatively common for one drug group to make a fake fire or ambulance call to a rival gang's turf in order to break up a drug deal. Sometimes, twitchy drug dealers would shoot at us when we knocked on the door, and ask questions later. So as we knocked, John and I did not stand in front of the door—we stood on either side of it so that any bullets that came flying out would miss us.

Today, however, there were no shots and we were let into a stuffy room that looked as if it had been hastily tidied. On the couch was a woman who was not moving and looking incredibly gray. On closer inspection, we found she was not breathing. I secured her airway and John worked her up as an unconscious-unknown patient. He started an IV with dextrose and immediately gave her the Narcan, a drug that counters the effects of an overdose. We were pretty sure she had done some drugs to cause this coma with respiratory arrest, and Narcan might bring her back. It did just that. She started breathing in a few seconds and woke up shortly thereafter. We were going to bring her to the ER to make sure the Narcan continued to work. The problem was, depending on the type of drug and how she took it, the Narcan could stop working after a while, and the OD could resume. However, Alice, our victim, came to and refused to go to the hospital. In fact, she was furious with us because we had ruined her trip. She started fighting to get out of the stretcher, pulled the IV out of her arm and proceeded to bleed all over us, the stretcher and the floor. We helped her out of the stretcher and made a quick retreat as she screamed at us for the waste of good drug money that we had caused her. Alice had wanted to party and we (with the help of the Narcan) had interfered.

Alice continued to party. We were called to her second party at about 3 a.m. and found her in the same condition: respiratory arrest. This time, John and I were able to get her to the hospital before she came around. In the ER, Alice hurled more epithets at the ER personnel for ruining her trip and wasting her money. For John and I it was déjà vu, and we briefed the ER staff on Alice's previous performance. Alice left the hospital against medical advice, hopefully to sleep it off. It's not every day that a person goes into respiratory arrest and is brought back twice.

We were called next to the bedroom of a well-kept house, where we were greeted by hysterical parents imploring us to help their son. In a macabre bedroom on the second floor was a well-built adolescent with a needle still sticking out of his arm, as though he had been suspended in time as he was injecting his street drug. The motionless teen, named Rob, had overdosed on heroin. While the police were managing the parents, John and I worked our patient and did a full code. Nonetheless, Rob died. Later in the hospital John seemed to have been fed up with ODs and drug abuse.

"Why try to escape reality?" he asked.

"Drugs are for those who can't handle reality, and reality is for those who cannot handle drugs," I said. "For me, I can't handle drugs."

On Saturday afternoon it was déjà vu all over again with Alice. She was in the same clothes, in respiratory arrest again. Her arms looked like a road map to a pimple convention, with track marks all up and down them. This created a problem because her arms were so full of track marks that we couldn't get an IV line started. Therefore, we intubated her to help her breathe, scooped her up and headed to the ER. In the ER, they needed to do a "cut down"—which means cutting into the skin with a scalpel to access a vein deep within the arm—then gave her Narcan and brought her back from yet another lethal OD. She was pretty weak from the heavy partying she had done that weekend, but Alice was still determined to leave the hospital and get back to tripping. The ER physician tried to admit her as a psych patient with the diagnosis of PFN (plain fucking nuts), but Alice got out of the hospital—against medical advice again—that afternoon. Before she made her ignominious exit, Alice knocked her stretcher to the ground and threw an IV tray (with lots of needles) at a technician. She also threatened the physician treating her and tried to claw one of the ER nurses. They had saved Alice's life and she repaid them with violence and disdain.

John and I had saved Alice's life three times in two days. For me, that was quite a roller coaster emotionally. Alice's behavior had become destructive, and when we were called to yet another drug house at 1 a.m. Sunday morning, we found her yet again. This time not only was she not breathing, but she had no pulse. John and I ran a full code on her all the way to the hospital. It was almost like a sick game to see if we could save the same person four times in one weekend. Alice's previous trips to the ER had made her a bit of a legend.

We did not save Alice from that last trip. She had used and abused the emergency services to an extreme that Labor Day weekend. In three days, she had attacked and maligned numerous ER and ambulance staff, and I have to say we were not sad to see her go. When the physician running the code called it to pronounce her time of death several people were heard to express relief that Alice was dead. We started off really wanting to save Alice, but she did not want to be saved. In her effort to reach some kind of high, she sent all of us on an emotional whirlwind. All our good work was wasted on someone who did not appreciate it or want it. Finally, she defied us to the ultimate and died in front of us. Even Holly, who saw life from a rosy perspective, conceded that death for Alice would put her in a better place. John said it would be better if Alice was in any place other than here.

This kind of emotional frustration is not uncommon in the emergency services of big cities. When people ask me if certain TV shows or movies are realistic, I always say that if they would portray the EMS staff as happy or relieved when a subab dies, and in a way that made the audience agree with that sentiment, then I would consider these shows an accurate reflection of life on the job.

The following week, while studying for the tests I needed to pass to get into medical school, I continued to fret over Alice and our failed efforts to save her. The training and experience of a host of skilled people had no benefit for Alice. It made me reflect on the life of a physician. As I had learned from spending time with the pre-med students, most doctors went to medical school to help people. That's what I wanted, too. But would I be able to help people like Alice?

As I thought about this, I realized that a successful physician could treat only one patient at a time. This meant that the average physician really only helped a few thousand people in his or her career. I wanted to do more. I wanted to help people, but a *lot* of people. One patient at a time was too slow, especially in light of the fact that many people did not want to be helped or could not be helped by their physicians. This included not only Alice, but the smoker with lung cancer and the alcoholic with a failing liver. After much soul searching, I decided on a change of career path: my goal was to earn a doctorate and do research into the cause and treatment of diseases. Scientists like Sir Alexander Fleming, who discovered penicillin, and Albert Sabin, who developed the oral polio vaccine, helped *millions* of people. So would a researcher who could find a cure for cancer or a way to treat heart attack or stroke.

I cancelled my plans to attend medical school and signed up to take the entrance exams for graduate school. I was going to be a doctor, but one who would help people through research.

Visiting the Newborns

Medical and ambulance personnel are required to continuously update and practice their skills. Experience and training are keys to the job. We all did a variety of things to recertify ourselves and keep current in the latest techniques. This included specialized courses, participating in drills and reading EMS magazines. Knowledge and information made us better equipped to deal with what was thrown at us.

One summer I attended a training session on dealing with psychological emergencies. This included instruction on non-threatening behavior when dealing with violent or PFN patients, including a reminder to "get soft," so the patient can't use your pencil or anything else as a weapon. They also advised us that dress ties (as worn by some crews) had to be clip-on or violent patients could grab them and use them choke us.

This training session ended with something I didn't expect. The instructor wanted to know and discuss our personal techniques for dealing with the stresses of the job. This part of the class was definitely not on the syllabus. The instructor explained some of the usual techniques for this—things like sick jokes, denial and justification of the things we did and witnessed. Then there was the escapism of the people who might drink or party too hard when off the job. The instructor, Dr. Daniels, emphasized the importance of talking with colleagues and loved ones and reminded us that she was always available to talk with EMS personnel.

After the class, Steve Estes asked me, "What did you think of the shrink?" I knew he was referring to her looks, and she was attractive, but I said I didn't learn anything new from her talk because I was forever being analyzed by my psychology-major friends at college. They always wanted to know about the psych patients I had to deal with so they could play doctor and diagnose their conditions. These conversations always led to how this all made me feel. So I used a classic psych technique against them and went on the offensive by accusing them of going into psychology to solve their own problems. After that they usually left me alone—either because my attacks rang true or because they sensed that I wasn't open to their probing. Maybe some of what they were saying was true, but then again, I was living a double life.

News crews sometimes wanted to interview us on the ambulance and ride along to get footage of life and death on the streets. I was working with Bill once when we were assigned a newspaper reporter and his camera. This guy rode with us the whole day and every second we were not on a call he was asking us questions and taking pictures and video. Somehow, in the course of our endless conversations it came out that Bill and I had attended a coping course with Dr. Daniels and he wanted to know all about it. When the subject of how we deal with the job came up he asked me the classic question: "What do you do when you see something really bad?"

That was the question I was dreading. Fortunately, I was also prepared for it, and more at ease in this three-some situation to give my answer. "Simple," I said. "I go up to the third floor of the hospital where Obstetrics and Gynecology is and look at the new babies."

Bill didn't say a word—he had never known where I went on those occasions. The reporter just nodded while a silly grin formed on Bill's face.

Two days later, the quote was in the newspapers. Two days and thirty seconds later, Dr. Daniels asked to see me the next time I worked a day shift. I agreed and during the next two night shifts I also made my pilgrimage to Obstetrics and Gynecology to watch the newborns. One of these shifts was on a stifling hot summer evening. The windows in the ambulance were down and we had the police radio as low as possible while Bill and I chatted about our experiences with the reporter the day before. We were just cruising around between calls in no-man's land when we heard three gunshots and saw a crowd gathering about 800 feet behind us. Several people were waving, and a couple were frantically running towards us. Bill was driving and he made no move to turn around or head to the scene. I was happy with his decision because there was no way we were going to be the first to arrive at a shooting in no-man's land. We heard the call for the ambulance and police, and two cars, a street crime unit, and a motorcycle were dispatched to the scene immediately. A police car was soon coming down the street in the direction of the shooting with lights and sirens on. So we hit the lights and sirens too, and turned around to put ourselves right behind the police car. As we were turning, some of the people who had been running to get our attention reached the ambulance out of breath and shouted that there was a shooting. I tried to look surprised and said thanks for the information.

We got to the scene with the lead cruiser, which was driven by a rookie cop named Ron. He was a very young guy with red hair and freckles. Bill and I got the equipment and arrived at the side of the victim, who turned out to be a prominent Homme gang member, just as the rookie was about to start mouth-to-mouth. I asked Ron to back off, because I needed to intubate the victim. This would supply the victim with 100 percent oxygen while the rookie's lungs could only supply 20 percent. However, a fellow gang member of the victim who heard this exchange didn't know about the difference in oxygen-delivering capacity and immediately started to throw accusations at us.

"What's the matter? Ain't you going to save the brother?" he screamed. The Hommes accumulating around the scene (who could be recognized by the colors they wore) were a close-knit group and this particular agitator seemed to command a lot of respect. More people arrived, and accusations of racism began flying at Ron the rookie and at Bill and me. We were all white and at the scene with a mortally wounded Homme in the heart of Homme territory. Two other cops arrived (one black and one white) and they called for backup, ordering the rookie, Bill, and me out of the scene. Bill and I did not even have a chance to intubate the victim—we just whisked him off to the hospital. Unfortunately, the damage had been done in the heart of Homme turf, and both the tension and the number of Homme members continued to build. Within 20 minutes the area was declared a riot scene and the police and EMS were mobilized. Bill, Ron and I were sequestered for the rest of the evening and interviewed by a couple of detectives. The detectives also gave us news reports on the progress of the riot we had caused. I wasn't sure if they did this as a way of chastising us for what we had done or if they just wanted to keep us informed.

Fortunately, no one was seriously injured during this mini riot on Homme turf. The papers said that a drug-related shooting sparked a riot. Thank God for the papers not getting the full story again. Though the detectives and my colleagues all agreed that it was no one's fault, this event did cause me to make a visit to Obstetrics and Gynecology that night—pilgrimage number one.

Two days after the reporter rode with us, Bill and I had a "woman in labor" call. I had been on lots of these, and they usually meant that the woman's spouse or partner was not available to drive her to the hospital. So we were just a big taxicab with expensive equipment. I had never actually caught the kid and did not expect to today. But this time Bill and I did assist a woman in delivering and Bill caught the baby girl. Immediately after, I was rummaging through the childbirth supply pack for the clamps to tie off the cord. The placenta would be coming out soon and we needed to cut the cord, but where were the clamps? Bill insisted I find something he could use to tie off the cord. I had to improvise, so I took off my shoelaces and handed them to Bill. That ambulance contained about $50,000 in medical equipment and I had to sacrifice my shoelaces for this woman's newborn. Later that day, I went up to Obstetrics and Gynecology to see the little girl that Bill and I helped bring into this world. It was one of the very few times I ever went to the viewing area when I wasn't depressed. I went there happy and left happier.

When Dr. Daniels finally ushered me into her office the next day, she said she supported my visits to the newborns, but cautioned that one should have more permanent methods for dealing with these stresses. She asked me when was the last time I visited the viewing area and whether the visits getting more frequent. I suppressed a chuckle and against my better judgment told her the truth. I admitted I had been there twice in the last two days, and told her why. I also described our experiences with the reporter, and by the end of our little meeting Dr. Daniels was convinced I should stay in college. She felt that college would make me a more valuable employee and better able to deal with the stresses of the job. I had no doubt that superior training would make me better at the job, but I was worried about what the job might make me become.

When I reported my conversation with Dr. Daniels to Holly, she suggested I continue working on the ambulance while going to college. With a degree, I could do whatever I wanted on the ambulance. The problem was that I sometimes felt that the stuff in college was puerile and parochial, with no semblance of real life involved, whereas the ambulance *was* real life, albeit a harsh side of it. I tended to use one as an escape from the other. This formed a kind of balanced schizophrenia for me, which I realized while talking to Holly.

I listened to Holly's suggestion and stayed in college.

Drunks Are a Part of the Job

There is an old saying among EMS personnel that if you are at a single-car accident after 2 a.m. and you haven't found a drunk, then keep looking. Drunks cause lots of car accidents, of course. But they also get hurt in more interesting ways.

Paul Weinstein, my partner for this shift, was one of the smartest guys on the ambulance. He was the son of one of the ER physicians, and everyone who knew him thought he should become a physician too. He was an excellent paramedic and his patients were all made to feel comfortable and safe. He was distinguished looking and had a British accent that made him sound even more intelligent. Even in a dirty ambulance uniform, he was the picture of a professional.

It was a Friday night and the full moon was keeping the streets illuminated better than the 60-year-old streetlights. Paul and I were called to a scene where a person was in police custody. The police wanted us to take their suspect, who had several injuries, to the ER. They had gone to an address in a housing project to arrest some guy who, they soon discovered, was drunk and had started a fight in the street with the neighbors. He fled into the apartment building and numerous witnesses told police where he could be found. These witnesses also said that the drunk had flashed a knife, but the descriptions were vague and they varied from witness to witness. In this neighborhood, it was unusual to get so much information from the local people, so the cops were surprised by the assistance they were receiving. Most of the witnesses were drunk too, which partially explained their willingness to talk.

This building was six stories high and our call was on the top floor. Moreover, the elevators were out— as usual. When we arrived, Paul grabbed the trauma kit and I brought the stair chair and we both started the long climb up the stairs. (The stair chair is a piece of equipment that enabled us to carry a patient down stairs safely and efficiently.) We were met at about the fourth floor by the police, who had been gracious and considerate enough to start walking the drunk down the stairs. As they approached us, one of the cops advised us that the victim claimed to have been pushed down the stairs by the people outside and that this had caused various injuries to his head. This was also the way the fight started. The police officer ended his brief with a sarcastic tone: "I'm not really sure how he got the cut on his head."

Well, our drunk was aware enough to know he was being belittled and proceeded to demonstrate to us what had happened. "You see," he slurred, "they pushed me from behind and I went like this…" Now the drunken gentleman lunged forward, trying to look like he had been pushed from behind. With his hands handcuffed behind his back, however, he had no way to stop himself, and he simply rolled down the stairs. He gained speed as he rolled toward where Paul and I were standing below. His screams and grunts increased as he got closer to us. Paul was behind me and he ran around the corner to the next landing, while I was still in the path of the rapidly rolling drunk. The cops and Paul were yelling to me to get out of the way, but there wasn't enough time. So, still holding the stair chair, I grabbed the banisters on both sides of the narrow stairs and lifted my legs up off the steps to let the out-of-control drunk roll underneath me.

Paul peeked his head around the corner and laughed. "Hey, I didn't know you were part Spiderman," he yelled up to me. The cops thought my little gymnastics trick was quite funny, too. Now, however, Paul and I had a real call. The drunk had a couple more cuts added to the original cut on his head, was unconscious, and had an obviously fractured right arm as well as a rigid abdomen, a sign of intestinal injury or internal bleeding. The fact that it became rigid so fast was an ominous sign.

Transferring the patient to the stretcher while in the stairwell was problematic. We got the stretcher as close as possible, but then decided to carry him out of the stairway. Normally, when lifting a patient, one person would grab the legs at the knees and the other person would pass their arms under armpits of the victim and then grab his own wrists. Thus the patient's arms would be crossed and he or she could be lifted easily. Since this patient was handcuffed and the cop would not uncuff him, however, all I could do was get behind him and grab him just under his armpits. Despite the difficulties and cramped space, we got him on the stretcher and to the hospital.

Paul and I had to make a statement to the police to verify that the injuries the man sustained while in police custody were his own fault. There was a special report that needed to be filled out, and in a tiny little box it said, "What was the cause of the injury?" My answer: "Stupidity."

The patient on our next call looked remarkably like the previous one. He was in his mid-20s and also quite intoxicated. This patient, however, was in bed—the top bunk of a bunk bed. How he came to have a broken arm and a severely bruised face and abdomen was a mystery. He was semi-conscious and not too coherent. There were about 10 intoxicated friends at hand helping to confuse things. We learned that the group was part of a basketball team and they had been celebrating a big win. Our victim, Tim, had passed out in the midst of the group, so he was hoisted on the shoulders of some friends and thrown into the bunk bed. A few minutes later, while the friends were busy partying,

Tim knocked on the door. Not knowing how he had
managed to go outside, the whole team brought him
back upstairs and threw him into bed again, admonish-
ing him for going outside. A few minutes later, Tim
walked in again and the group again picked him up and
started to bring him back up to the bunk bed. This time
they heard him whimper, "Guys, please don't throw
me out the window again." The top bunk, it turned out,
was right next to an open window, and the drunken
team members didn't realize that Tim was injured
when he came back into the house.

We got Tim to the hospital and even before we finished
giving our report to the Holly in the ED, we got a "man
down" call. A street person with a notorious drinking
history was seen shuffling across the street with that
familiar hunched-over walk. Suddenly he stopped in
mid-stride and fell face first to the pavement. According
to witnesses, he made no attempt to catch himself as he
fell and planted his chin directly on the pavement. The
result was that he was bleeding from the mouth and
had a bad laceration on his chin. Cuts to the face bleed
profusely and when people are loaded with alcohol they
can bleed even more heavily. So this drunk had a big
blood puddle around him, and he hadn't moved from
the spot where he had tasted the pavement. When I got
to him, Mr. Barker was in an obvious stupor, but it was
difficult to determine if this was from "kissing Ethyl" or
if he had a legitimate head injury.

As I talked with Mr. Barker to determine the extent
of his injuries, I noticed the extensive scarring on his

face. Chronic alcoholics accumulate scars and injuries as part of the lifestyle. They will drink, get very drunk, fall down and get a KON–LAC (laceration from a knock on the nut). Today Mr. Barker had added another pothole to his weatherworn face.

"Are you in any pain?" I enquired.

"My dentures!" he stammered through a toothless grimace.

"You don't have any teeth."

"My dentures don't fit right," he insisted.

"You don't have any dentures in."

"My dentures hurt," was the slurred response.

When people are injured, they frequently fixate on something. Dr. Daniels would explain that such patients are compensating and dissociating. A person with a broken arm might be concerned that her watch was broken or that a fingernail was broken. They distract themselves with some seemingly unimportant object as a way of ignoring their serious injuries. Nonetheless, I looked around the scene to see if there were any dentures on the ground. But I saw none. I thought about searching him for dentures, but decided against it. Rummaging around in someone's pockets could bring with it accusations of trying to rob the person or surprises that are too disgusting to mention. I wondered if there might be some problem with his jaw that might cause this fixation with the dentures he did not have in his mouth. I looked at Mr. Barker's scar-riddled face and noticed that his jaw was not hanging right. I asked him to open his mouth as wide as possible and when he tried, there was an extra bump on his chin. The chin-first fall to the pavement seemed to have broken his jaw and displaced it to the side a bit.

A broken jaw is very painful, but with the amount of alcohol Mr. Barker had in his bloodstream (0.34 percent blood alcohol, about four times the legal limit), he was very well anaesthetized. He did feel some pain, but only to the extent that it felt like his dentures did not fit. We brought him to the ER and advised them of the situation. An x-ray confirmed the break and Mr. Barker had his jaw wired shut for a few weeks. Paul commented that he would need to have his meals through a straw for that time, but this would not be new for Mr. Barker, because he got most of his meals from a straw sticking out of a brown bag.

We were not even finished getting Mr. Barker off the stretcher when we had another call. Our patient was a WT with the physique of a professional weightlifter and all the marks of a prominent gang member. He was also very drunk and decided that he wanted to show how tough he was. To do this, he hit himself on the head with a beer bottle. The bottle didn't break the first time he smashed it against his head, so according to witnesses he started to pound the right side of his head with it—wham, wham, wham against his head until the bottle finally broke. It was now razor sharp, but he continued to smash it against the side of his head. The result was multiple parallel LACs four to five inches long, from his lower jaw to the top of his temple. One cut just missed his right eye. It was out of character for any WT to call the ambulance, but someone did, and they even walked their drunk and delinquent gang member to the front yard and had him wait for us. Because it was risky territory and the partygoers inside the house were likely to have more weapons than the police, we picked up the WT without asking any questions and headed to the ED.

The ED was exceptionally busy, and Paul and I needed to catch up on some paperwork, so we decided to stay there for a while. Just then, Dr. Frank came in saying that she wanted to get going on suturing the WT. The nurse, Carol, left to get the suture tray. Dr. Frank was on the other side of the stretcher with the WT between her and me, and I started to brief her on the patient's slashes, and how they were "accidentally self-inflicted." Dr. Frank had the WT turn his head in her direction as she looked at his wounds, and in an absent-minded tone said, "That wasn't very bright, was it?"

The WT, his manly ego bruised, took offence at her comment and, seemingly from nowhere, produced a switchblade and thrust it towards Dr. Frank. I had brought this dangerous WT into the ER and felt somewhat responsible for what he was about to do, so I grabbed for the knife. Actually, I grabbed his wrist with both of my hands, and rolled his forearm down and away from Dr. Frank. Then, without thinking, I put all my weight on this guy's arm and smashed it onto the side of the stretcher. My intention was to make him let go of the knife. He did release the knife, but much to my surprise, I also broke his wrist. This all took about three seconds, and Dr. Frank did not make a sound. She simply looked me and then her eyes fell to the freshly broken wrist of the WT and she shook her head.

I have to admit that the rest of the incident is pretty much a blur. The WT started screaming from the pain, but this sounded distant to me because I was somewhat in shock over what had happened. I guess Dr. Daniels would say that I was compensating and dissociating. Carol picked up the knife and disposed of it, and security soon arrived. Dr. Frank and the ER nurse both advised security that the WT came in with a broken arm and the WT was sutured, casted and sent home. Carol and Dr. Frank seemed to silently agree to cover for me in that way.

Breaking that guy's arm was something that I did as a reflex. A few days later, a local detective asked me about the incident. The WT had discussed it with his attorney, and according to Tom the detective, the lawyer advised the WT that he was lucky not to have been charged with menacing and attempted assault with a deadly weapon. Tom also said that I actually could be eligible for an award for defending Dr. Frank. I told him there was nothing I wanted to recall about that incident. Neither Dr. Frank nor Carol ever talked to me about what had happened, but they lied to protect me and I appreciated their effort.

Since then I have run through the event many times in my head. I can feel and hear the bones breaking under my weight and hear the WT's cries of pain. I actually get angry with the WT for making me feel this way. I didn't intend to break his arm; I only wanted to prevent Dr. Frank from being injured. I am haunted by the thought of what would have happened if I hadn't stopped the WT. Might Dr. Frank have been killed? To this day, this is one event in my life that I wish had never happened. I wonder what Dr. Daniels would say about that.

Along for the Ride

Sometimes having a third person on the ambulance can be a big help and sometimes it is a huge liability. There were lots of people who spent time on the ambulance for various reasons. Sometimes cops who wanted to be certified as emergency medical technicians would ride with us for a while. Some police forces would give officers a raise for this certification or give them special assignments where those skills could be used—for example, the police who responded to car accidents with injuries would have EMT training. Trainee cops, trainee physicians, and nurses also regularly rode along with the ambulance crew. We even had ER intards ride with us to see what it was like in the streets. They sometimes had a hard time understanding that the ambulance is very different from ER. On the ambulance, normally there are only two people. Both must be willing and prepared to deal with almost anything.

We cannot pick and choose calls, nor can we easily call for quick help if we get stuck.

Everyone has aversions of some kind. Many people are afraid of heights or are claustrophobic, for example, and EMS personnel have their own phobias. Monica was a nurse in the ER who was extremely competent with anything you could throw at her, but she couldn't stand patients with severe bloody noses. When a person has a severe bloody nose, the blood clots come out as semisolid chunks, and this revolted Monica. Most of her fellow nurses would actually volunteer for the nosebleed cases before Monica would even get to the patient's chart.

Not so on the ambulance; we couldn't turn over patients to others. If there was a patient or condition we did not like to deal with, simply getting on with it was the only option. Even when an intard rode with us.

Paul and I we were carrying a third man on the ambulance one day, and he was trying very hard to impress us with his knowledge. He was actually a resident in internal medicine, not an intern. Nonetheless, to us he was an intard. He looked as if he should have been on a safari—the vest he was wearing had more pockets than a pool table. After medical school and some time in a successful residency, he felt that he had seen everything there was to see in medicine and had so much worldly experience that this ambulance stuff was going to be a breezy little diversion. It was surely going to be better than being constantly hounded by the people in the hospital. "There I would have to do real work," he said. To Paul and me, this implied that ambulance work was not real work. This was going to be a fun shift.

Our first call turned out to be trial by fire for us as well as for the intard. Fortunately, there was no actual fire, but the intard tried hard to kill himself.

We were dispatched to a multi-car accident with PI. A big silver Cadillac had rolled over and was sitting on its hood with the back end sticking up in the air. How did this happen on a straight stretch of road, I wondered to myself. There was something else about the scene that seemed wrong, though I couldn't pinpoint it. I knew we would want the fire department here. They weren't on scene yet, but they were close—I could hear their sirens in the distance.

In the Cadillac was a middle-aged man in a business suit, unconscious and hanging from his seat belt. The intard was out of the ambulance and racing to the car before Paul or I could get any equipment. As the intard scurried toward the car, I realized what was bothering me. This car was not well balanced in that position; it seemed likely to shift. I was pretty sure that the intard was going to do something gung-ho and stupid, so I grabbed our gear and ran after him. As I got close I also noticed another problem: the Cadillac was still running. It is very hard for a car to stay running following a flip—in fact, most mechanics say it is impossible, but I saw the back wheels of this vehicle turning.

The intard proceeded to do what some textbook lecturer had taught EMS people to do with unconscious victims trapped in cars. That is, get in the back of the car and check vitals while maintaining neck traction. This kind of treatment for a car accident victim is great, but it assumes that the car is still on its wheels. The intard was experiencing our old friend tunnel vision. He was so focused on the patient that he wasn't considering the surroundings. Getting into an overturned car is not safe for the uninitiated, and you should only do it with your eyes wide open. But before I could stop him, the intard began yanking on the back door to open it. This shifted the balance of the car and caused it to rock off the hood and back onto its roof. Interestingly, when this happened the engine finally stalled.

Realizing that he should have waited for us to secure the car and that the shift in position could have further injured the victim inside, the intard turned pale and looked at me fearfully. I wanted badly to reprimand him, but somewhere I felt some sympathy (and didn't want to sour the rest of the day), so I said, "I've never seen a car's engine turned off that way, but I'm glad it's not running anymore." He didn't look too relieved, but nodded an acknowledgement and we continued. Fortunately, the fire department arrived about then and we requested that the car be secured so I could crawl in and treat the patient.

The three of us never discussed the Cadillac seesaw that day. My hope was that the intard had learned that EMS in the streets required more than simply knowing how to treat patients—such as what can get you killed and how to avoid that.

The next call came in simply as "ambulance requested" and gave absolutely no details. The address was a very dangerous part of town, which meant that the ambulance would normally be supplied with police backup. But dispatch was not sending anyone to accompany us.

The address we'd been called to was on the fourth floor of an apartment building, at the far end of a hall. Paul and I stood to the right of the big door and knocked. It's dangerous to stand immediately in front of a door because you never know what can come out of it, such as a fleeing perpetrator or even bullets. So SOP required that we stand to the side of a door, knock, and yell "Ambulance!" Paul was knocking and we both were yelling when I noticed the heavy hinges on the door. This was some secure apartment. I also became aware that the intard was not next to me, but in front of the door. Without a word, I grabbed the back of his shirt and pulled him against the wall next to me. At that same moment, this huge door flew open. If the intard had not moved, he would have been knocked flat on his ass because the door swung out. There was another door behind that one that opened into the apartment. Again, there was some serious security in this apartment. Standing there was an intimidating looking WT who completely filled the doorway. Behind him, I could see his backup: two fellow gang members who were not doing a very good job of concealing their weapons.

"We didn't order no ambulance," the head man informed us, as I watched the two guys behind him for signs of weapons action. People doing drug deals get very protective of their territory during the deals. We had been sent to a drug house to break up a drug deal. This was a real bad situation.

From behind me came the words of a naive intard who was behaving like someone who wanted to get killed that day. "But we need to see if there is anyone injured in there."

This was absolutely the wrong thing to say. If these WTs thought we were going to try to force our way into their drug dealing apartment, they would change our minds with some "ballistic attitude adjustment."

"No, we don't," Paul quickly corrected. "False alarm. Sorry." As he began backing up, I pushed the intard out of my way and backed away slowly, too. The WT slammed the door and we retreated to the relative safety of our ambulance. Back at the ambulance I began screaming at the intard. "I don't care if you get yourself killed, but don't take us with you. So *please* keep your mouth shut!"

For the next two hours, Paul and I educated this intard further on the simple philosophy of the EMS people on the streets. The watchword is survival and you do nothing that will risk this. You especially do nothing to risk the survival of others around you. We forcefully pointed out that in two calls he had taken himself and us to the brink of becoming death statistics. We did not want a medal for heroism and we especially did not want a monument. Even though he had an MD, he was not streetwise and he needed to shut up and learn. We reminded him that the third man on the ambulance is there to observe.

Dr. Intard became very annoyed with our diatribes and informed us that he was the most educated in the group and that he was there to experience medicine in the streets, and that we had nothing to teach him. For him, the streets were a fishbowl he could watch from the safety of his protected world. We, however, were the fish in that bowl, where things can get stirred up in wild ways. "I am a medical doctor with eight years of college," he continued. "I don't need to know which gang fights with its neighbors." His defense was sounding a lot like a whiny kid trying to convince us his mommy said he could. It was pathetic.

The rest of the day was largely uneventful. Paul and I were catching up on what we hoped would be the last of the paperwork and the intard was trying to impress one of the ER nurses with his exploits during his single day in the streets. (I would later entertain Holly with an account of the intard's actions.) Suddenly, Paul marched up to the intard with the police radio in hand and said, "Time to make like a carrot." Holly and I knew what he meant, but the intard had a blank look on his face.

"What does that mean?"

"We've got a call, so we have make like a carrot and be 'on root.'"

Off we went to a cardiac arrest in a crowded restaurant. There were tons of people around, and a very large man in a business suit was on his back with an even larger woman thumping on his chest, trying to do CPR.

Paul advised her to continue as the three of us set things up. Paul intubated, I set up the EKG monitor and started recording, and the intard started an IV in our victim's left arm. He got the IV in on the first try and held the bag up high like a trophy. The code was actually working quite well when the intard decided it was his place to direct Paul and me. He had unilaterally decided to run the code and started telling us what to do. What he was directing us to do was all good medical practice, but he could have helped us do some of the procedures. He didn't do anything himself except hold the IV bag and give orders.

The EKG monitor showed ventricular fibrillation, so the intard told Paul to defibrillate. Paul gelled the paddles, placed them on the victim's bare chest, and yelled "clear." This was my cue to scan the floor—you don't want anyone to be kneeling or standing in water or urine, or that person can receive a massive shock. You also had to make sure that you were electrically disconnected from the patient before shouting "clear." However, the intard, who was still standing by the patient's head, yelled "clear" even though he was holding on to the IV bag. So Paul defibrillated the patient. This had the desired effect: it brought back an acceptable heart rhythm and pulse. But the electrical current traveled up the IV solution and gave the intard a tremendous shock, which sent him to the floor. The intard, who had been showing off for the restaurant crowd, was now twitching with violent muscle contractions caused by a defibrillation he had ordered and cleared.

I drove the ambulance to the hospital and the intard was in the back with Paul. Paul told me later that the intard begged us to not write him up and to keep this story a secret. It hasn't been told until now, so I guess we kept our bargain. I felt at the time that this was a case of mutual protection. We could have gotten in trouble for not making him get rid of the IV bag, and he could have been in trouble for not clearing when he called clear. That was the last call of the day and the intard disappeared from the ER immediately after we transferred our heart attack patient to the ED staff.

In the weeks that followed, when we passed the intard in the halls, he never acknowledged Paul or me. He also never rode on an ambulance again.

Brothers in Arms

One evening, my partner Tom and I had a special guest on the ambulance, a police officer who was interested in doing some EMS time. He was my brother Jim.

Our first call that night was an elderly woman who was having "a spell" according to her daughter. This was no obvious medical emergency (it was an LOL in NAD), but her daughter said that her mother's spells could progress to epileptic seizures—she called them "letric scissors." She said that once a seizure started it was too hard to move her, so she wanted the ambulance to take her mother to the hospital immediately.

The mother had begun to "peripheralize," or use the muscles on only one side of her body, which was consistent with an impending seizure. She was hardly using her left side at all, and as she stepped forward with her right leg, dragging her left leg along, she was literally walking in circles. Jim stared in amazement at this woman slowly circling her way to the ambulance. None of us had ever seen anything like this, and it was sadly entertaining. I wanted to talk to one of the neurosurgery intards to see how it could be explained. She did not have a seizure during the ride to the ambulance and was transferred to the ER without incident.

We were called next to a low-income housing project where Richie in dispatch said "officer needs assistance." A single officer had been sent to the residence because the neighbors had not seen the occupant of one of the apartments for several days. The landlord had not received the most recent rent check and could not make contact with the elderly woman who lived in the apartment. So the police and building superintendent were going to enter the apartment with the passkey and break the chain if necessary. In view of the woman's prolonged absence, they fully expected to find a dead person in the apartment. The ripe odor of decomposing flesh told them that they were not likely to be disappointed. There were several neighbors and rubber-neckers in front of the door as the super used his key to open it. He and the cop then took deep breaths and entered. As soon as they went in, a neighbor disgusted by the smell closed the door behind them.

Inside they were confronted with a severely decomposed body, complete with maggots, insects, rats and other vermin feasting on the body. The smell was concentrated in the apartment because all the windows and doors were sealed tight. There had been so much decomposition in the room that all the oxygen had probably also been consumed. Because I was a chemistry major, I knew the oxygen in the air would be converted to carbon dioxide and methane gas as the woman's body decayed. Therefore, there would be very little oxygen for the PO and superintendent to breathe. This woman may have once been young, beautiful, charming and intelligent. But after death her body succumbed to the natural processes of biology and chemistry. The result was unrecognizable blob of flesh, fluid, and exposed bone that was once a human being.

The combination of sights, smells and the lack of oxygen caused both the cop and the super to pass out. Fortunately, because methane gas is lighter than oxygen, there was enough O_2 at floor level for the PO to regain consciousness and call for help on the radio. He then crawled across the floor, dragging the superintendent with him, opened the door of the apartment and closed it behind him.

We arrived to find a groggy PO and an angry superintendent. "Who told you to close the door?" he yelled at the neighbor. Our arrival distracted the superintendent just long enough for the neighbor to scurry off.

We gave them both oxygen and attempted to re-enter the apartment. There was nothing we could do, but my brother wanted to see the body. The smell outside the apartment was impossible to describe. The projects always smelled like sweat, urine and feces, but the stench of a decaying body is a distinctly disgusting one. Like the PO and superintendent, we took deep breaths and went in. We saw a woman who had literally melted into her couch. There were so many maggots and other creatures in and on her body that it looked as if her clothes and skin were moving. We were in the apartment only as long as we could hold our breaths, and when we went back outside it was unanimously agreed that the FD would have to move the body. The FD eventually entered the apartment with breathing apparatus, a body bag and shovels. They shoveled as much of the corpse as they could into the body bag and turned it over to the ME. The ME had a special room for doing an autopsy on a corpse like this. It was a "wind tunnel" where air would be blown continuously over the body and then out a vent. The ME would work on the upwind side of the tunnel so as not to be overcome by the smell. Neither the PO nor the superintendent needed to go to the hospital, so we left the scene and went back in service.

Our next call was a classic PFN patient. We were called to a "domestic dispute," and two police cars were dispatched along with us. As the story went, a woman called the police to report that her husband had come home and killed her. When she called 911 she had actually said, "I'm dead. He killed me." You can see how this can be a complicated situation. A woman is claiming to have a homicidal husband, while also informing dispatch of her own death. Who is the crazy person here?

When we arrived at the scene, the woman ran frantically out of the house towards us. It was a cool summer evening, and she was wearing pink flannel pajamas and what looked like a blue hospital gown as a kind of robe. She screeched in a high-pitched voice that her husband claimed he was told by voices to kill her, but she convinced him that she was dead, so she was still alive. This little exchange told me that she was a psych patient, but we still needed to determine if there was some other danger in the house—the husband could be PFN, too. We asked her to take us to her husband, who was clearly visible through the big windows of the large two-story brick house, which had been built about the turn of the century, but was exceedingly well-kept inside and out. He was sitting in the living room, calmly watching TV.

Tom, Jim and I got soft and headed for the house, followed by the police. Cops don't like to get soft—they prefer to keep their weapons. We knocked and the husband came to the door. He regarded us with only slight surprise and asked, "What did she tell you to get you here this time?" I told him the story.

"Voices telling me to kill her is one of her better ones," he said with a slight smile. He went on to explain that his wife had suffered from mental illness for several years. She did not call 911 too often, he said, but the first time she called she had said that he was trying to kill her. Her story was so convincing that the police arrested him and he spent a night in jail. When she went to the police station to finish filing her complaint, she started to describe how the voices were really talking to her husband and the police eventually released him.

We did not bring the woman to the hospital. She was not a threat to herself or anyone else, and her husband promised to make an appointment for his wife to see the doctor the next morning.

Jim was shocked by the story we just heard. "Do you really think that anyone could have believed her and had the husband arrested?" He was disturbed to know that a PFN could make a claim against a sane spouse, and have the spouse spend the night in jail.

"Yes," was my simple response. I knew it could happen if it was the first time, if the person was not so obviously disturbed and if the husband was too aggressive with his denials. Today he had stayed completely out of it, although he was probably upset with his wife. Realizing that we were assessing his mental state, he was exceedingly calm and rational. He'd been through this before and learned a lesson. "Imagine how you would respond if I suddenly claimed *you* were crazy. You would vehemently deny it and any hint of a loss of control could be interpreted as mental imbalance."

My brother was not comfortable with my assessment of this situation. As a PO, he was not ready to believe that the police could be so easily snowed by a psych patient. But anyone can be. For example, I had been dispatched a number of times to psych units containing violent offenders, either to pick someone up or drop them off. I had learned from the employees in these places that the only way to be sure who is the patient and who is the staff member is by checking to see if they have keys or ID badges.

We were dispatched next to a call of "man down," and the address was in no-man's land, in front of a block of housing projects between WT and Homme territories. We had almost reached the address when we were flagged down by at least 20 people in front of another notorious project, all of them in Homme colors.

"Yo, yo, yo, we called the ambulance," a prominent Homme wearing full colors informed Tom when we stopped. We were in an area known for dealing drugs, and the street and sidewalk were littered with broken glass, baggies and the vials often used for drug transactions.

"You called the ambulance?" I asked. "OK, what happened?" I hadn't moved from my seat and was not about to leave the safety of the ambulance until I got a fix on what was going on here.

"He hit the deck and got cut up, man," said the Homme as he pointed to a fellow gang member coming towards us with a couple of deep LACs on his hands and arms. With an obvious patient identified, I got out and brought the trauma kit with me. Tom parked the ambulance and was approached by another Homme with cuts on his arms. Jim was shadowing me and he was approached by a third person with cuts on her elbows and knees.

"Why do so many people have cuts?" I asked.

"When we heard the shots, we all hit the deck."

The word "shots" got my attention, and before I could even process the information, Tom was on the radio calling for multiple backup following a shooting in no-man's land. Thankfully, several police cars swiftly joined us and officers were soon interviewing the many witnesses. Apparently someone from the ARPs came along and opened fire. He missed everyone, but there were lots of people with cuts on their arms and legs because they all dropped to the ground as the shots rang out. All the injuries we had on that call were from people diving for cover, and none were gunshot wounds.

As we would treat the Hommes for minor cuts and LACs, they would be whisked off by the police to help them find the ARP shooter. The police would rather find the shooter this way than by having the Hommes try to punish the ARP. This process of "treat and retreat" continued until there were no more police cars and it was just me, Tom, my brother and a few uninjured Hommes. It is not the wisest thing to be in no-man's land immediately after a shooting, and be unarmed. I think all three of us had that same feeling of overwhelming vulnerability when Jim said, "My ankle is itching."

My brother the off-duty police officer had his service revolver holstered to his ankle and this was the signal to leave. But before we could go, dispatch called and advised us that the original "man down" was still waiting for us, two blocks away—some poor gentleman who had broken his arm in a fall.

So ended my brother's experience on the ambulance. It impressed him so much that he's now a lawyer. He claims the career change had nothing to do with the decomposing old lady or his itchy ankle.

Alternate Uses for the Ambulance

Sometimes I was lucky enough to be assigned a soft shift, and any assignment that was easy, or even just different, was always welcome. One of the more interesting of these was serving as standby at a university soccer game. A lot of sporting events are required to have an ambulance standby in case someone gets hurt and I got one of these shifts. It turned out that my own university's soccer team was in a local final. The coach was also a professor in the chemistry department, so I knew him pretty well. I also knew many of the team members.

Even though it was a final, there was not much of a crowd, because Division III college soccer is not a big draw. Still, it was an enjoyable way to spend an ambulance shift. The fans, myself included, were very into the game. Tom and I got to park the ambulance close to the field, so we had the best seat in the house. It was a cool autumn evening with a light rain. I didn't bring a raincoat and I wanted to stand on the sidelines with my friends on the team. (As a member of the safety personnel, I had that right and I was going to exercise it.) One of my friends gave me one of the team's spare raincoats, which made me look like one of the players standing on the sidelines.

It was a close, well played game and very physical. Because of the wet conditions there were a lot of sliding tackles from both teams, which is exciting as well as dangerous. Tension was getting pretty high as the teams were tied 2–2. An injury seemed all too likely, given the intensity of the game and the wet field conditions. I was caught up in the energy and excitement, but I was not anxious to bring someone to the hospital. Then one of the opposing defenders made a dangerous tackle. It happened just 10 feet in front of me, and I screamed at the referee that it was a dangerous play and that he should try to keep control of the game. I ran after the referee as I shouted at him.

The referee stopped play and started to take out the red card to kick me out of the game. I pulled off the raincoat to show him I was with the ambulance, not the team, and said, "If you make me leave, the game is over. You can't continue this game without the ambulance standing by. So, I guess it's your call."

The referee, frustrated and angry, replied, "Keep quiet or else you're out of here."

With that, the coach, my chemistry professor, got involved. "You can't dismiss him like that. He's here in compliance with NCAA regulations, and in his opinion you're allowing an unsafe level of play. If you ignore his advice and insist that he leave, I'll file a complaint with the NCAA. He's part of the safety personnel, so you can't ignore his opinion." The coach neglected to mention that I was a student in one of his classes, but perhaps that was best.

There was much snickering from the team as the disgruntled referee agreed to call any dangerous plays and skulked away. I was not kicked out of the game and we ended up winning. Not that I helped, but the team did seem much more motivated after the coach yelled at the referee. Moreover, I got an invitation to the team dinner at the end of the season and that little incident became a legend in the athletic department.

When the game was over, Tom and I wanted to stay on the clock for as long as possible. So we went to the ER, a safe haven where we could flirt with Holly, catch up on our paperwork and be available to jump any interesting calls.

Tom was filling out the run sheets and I was helping the ER staff with a Homme who had been brought in by another ambulance. This patient was semiconscious from a couple of GSWs to the abdomen. He was a huge man, with strikingly long and thick dreadlocks, a solid mass of muscle with scars all over his face, arms and chest. He may have been tattooed gangland-style. From the road map of crisscrossing scars, this guy must be a real street fighter. The ER staff stripped him and the cops went through his personal effects but, surprisingly, found no guns or other weapons. This was unusual for a gang member, but maybe his gun had been lost in the firefight. That however, was not our concern at this time. Giving him fluids and getting him up to the OR were the most urgent problems.

I noticed that the victim's head was propped up and forward due to his thick dreadlocks. Even though he did not seem to be having a problem breathing, it was best to make sure there was no obstruction to his airway. So I went to take care of this while the rest of the ER staff was focusing on his abdomen. I tried to move his dreadlocks out of the way and tilt his head back and just couldn't do it. I felt a huge knot of some sort in the hair at the very back of his head and tried to shift it to the right. To my surprise, the knot completely pulled away from his hair and I was left holding a .38 revolver. This Homme hid his gun in his hair. I told Holly to call hospital security, who turned the gun over to the police. I showed the cops the patch of hair that contained the gun and found some cloth strips that had been used to hold the weapon in place. One of the police sergeants wanted to take a picture of the gun hidden in the hair for training purposes, and he started to put the gun back. We insisted that if he wanted to replace the gun for a photo that the bullets had to be removed first, even if the patient was unconscious and restrained.

Later that evening, Tom and I grabbed a huge take-out dinner from an all-night diner and drove to the park with our feast. There was enough food for four people, but that was OK because sometimes we would nibble at a meal for hours. It was a beautiful clear summer evening and the park was a well known spot for high school kids to play in the back seats of cars or vans. Tom liked to entertain us by cruising the park in the ambulance and finding parked cars. He knew the parking places well, because he had done the same thing when he was younger. Tonight he seemed determined to get to a certain place quietly. He turned off all the lights and guided the ambulance with soft touches on the accelerator, stopping by using the emergency brake or the neutral gear so there would be no brake lights. Finally, he spotted a station wagon parked under some trees. "There it is!" It was backlit by the lights from the highway on the other side of the park, so we had a great view of the silhouettes in the car.

Tom turned to me and with a maniacal grin said, "That's my parent's car. My brother is on a date with his girlfriend and they're probably going at it hot and heavy inside."

With even greater caution and stealth, Tom inched the ambulance to within 10 feet of the car. The front of the ambulance was directly parallel with the wagon, and we could see bouncing up and down in the back seat. When the rhythm of the bouncing seemed to be reaching a crescendo Tom simultaneously turned on the headlights, emergency lights, and siren and yelled into the loudspeaker "Freeze—it's the pooooooooolice."

Two heads popped up inside the car with sheer terror in their eyes. Tom and I were laughing hysterically when his brother jumped half-naked out of the car and charged the ambulance. Meanwhile, the girl got out and ran toward the woods. Tom and his brother were having a major tiff, so they didn't see the girlfriend try to escape. I got their attention just as the shadowy form of a female disappeared into the woods. They headed into the woods to try and catch her, and I stayed with the ambulance (lights off now) in case she came back.

The three of them returned a short while later, and Tom and I shared the dinner we had brought. The girl's name was Sharon and she clung to Tim, Tom's brother, while we went through some uncomfortable introductions. They finally settled down and we had a pleasant little visit. She was a high school senior planning to go to a rival college to the one I attended. I told her a few things about college life and tried to not sound like I was pontificating. We also told them some ambulance stories, including the story of John and Jane Doe who had died in that same park. Sharon seemed a bit disconcerted by this story, but Tim tried to reassure her by saying that they were safe because the engine was not running. Tom broke the four of us up then by saying, "Yeah, but *your* motor was sure running when we pulled up."

The mood gradually began to lighten, and I went into the ambulance and turned on my little portable radio. I then switched on the PA system to activate the speaker and hooked the radio to the outside speaker. For the next half hour we ate dinner with Tim and Sharon and listened to the radio on the ambulance loudspeaker. Tom's brother and his girlfriend were a cute pair, and I wondered if Holly and I would make such a nice couple.

Speaking of Holly, the nursing students were going on a field trip to the Kissler Rehabilitation Institute. A world-renowned facility, Kissler was doing fantastic things for the treatment of those with debilitating injuries, especially head and neck injuries. I was interested in going, because I thought it would help me better understand these patients. We spent a relatively short time treating them, yet many needed years to recover from their injuries, and some never recovered. A person with a broken neck and spinal cord injury might be saved by our efforts, only to be relegated to life in a wheelchair with severe disabilities. I felt I needed be exposed to such things to understand the consequences of the part I was playing. Besides, Holly would be going.

I tried to get on the list without success. However, as luck would have it, the bus driver scheduled to take the students to Kissler was sick that day. The field trip organizers recalled my interest in going along and felt that a person experienced in driving an ambulance could drive a bus. So I was invited to be the driver and would be able to tour the facilities with the nurses.

Holly was surprised to see me behind the wheel of the bus when she got in, and quickly sat in the seat right behind me. However Nurse Rothchild deemed it necessary to sit near me to give directions to Kissler, so Holly moved back a few seats.

At Kissler we saw all sorts of different therapists treating a wide array of patients. Some patients were lacking limbs, others had withered limbs and were learning to use their feet as hands. Kissler also had an enormous amount of equipment for rehabilitation and research. A patient was encouraged to stay in the institute as long as he or she showed progress. That meant that if you stopped getting better you were discharged. It was a philosophy to inspire hard work by both patients and staff.

We saw patients who had had their legs amputated learning how to walk on new custom-made prosthetics. The staff explained that an amputation below the knee was "better" than one above the knee. (They used the terms BKA and AKA for below- and above-knee amputation.) When the knee was intact, the patient had better balance and mobility for controlling the prosthetic devices they were learning to walk with. Holly was especially interested in a 16-year-old girl who had lost her left foot and her right leg below the knee when she was hit by a drunk driver. The girl, whose name was Shelly, was learning to walk on two prosthetic devices designed specially for her. Shelly seemed to have good balance and a very positive attitude. She was especially eager to be able to wear a skirt to school. Amazingly, the color of the prosthetic devices matched the rest of her legs perfectly.

Holly chatted with the girl's mother about the accident. Apparently the driver was an alcoholic and subab with a long history of drunk driving. She had no insurance, had had her license revoked and was drinking at a bar where the bartender should have known she was too drunk to drive. This driver was now in jail and her two kids (who were usually left alone while their mother went to the bar) were in foster care. Shelly's mother was still disturbed by how many lives, including her daughter's and her own, were forever changed by the accident.

I stayed with Holly and listened to the story while I watched the therapist train Shelly to shift her hips to control the swing of her artificial legs, and to use her back and arms to keep her balance. These acrobatic motions were like a choreographed dance that Shelly used to walk, turn and manage stairs. Holly was visibly upset by the story and hung on Shelly's mother's every word.

While I saw many things that day for the first time, it was not my first visit to Kissler. Several years before, my cousin broke his neck in a diving accident that left him permanently paralyzed, with no use of his legs and limited use of his arms after fracturing the fourth and fifth vertebrae in his neck. I had visited him in Kissler and appreciated what the staff were doing for him. I knew that the rehabilitation was designed to optimize the function he had remaining, not to return function. My family was hoping for a better outcome, but he, like many victims of spinal cord injury, never regained normal use of his arms and legs.

Killing Time in the ER

Late one winter, when the weather was just starting to warm up, I was working in the ER rather than the ambulance because money was tight and the pay was slightly better. Sometimes, too, I would work in the ER between shifts because the ambulance was trying not to not schedule people for too many shifts in a row, in order to avoid liability from sleep-deprived staff.

When times were really tough, the ER was also a place where I could get free meals. Physicians would order special meals for certain patients in the ER, and I would usually be the one to go to the kitchen to pick up the trays. The request, for example, might be for "soft food, low sodium" for someone with bad teeth and a blood pressure problem. Because the majority of these meals were for indigent patients, the kitchen personnel would not even bother to do the paperwork for billing. So during the course of a shift, I would request a regular meal for "a poverty case in the ER" and eat it myself. I figured that I wasn't technically lying, because my income was definitely below the poverty level. This gave me the dubious distinction of being the only person I know who ever went out of his way to eat hospital food.

The ER was much more civilized and controlled than working on the streets, where anything could happen. However, the ER often required me to deal with a number of patients at once, as opposed to one at a time on the ambulance. I might be part of a team treating a patient with a laceration, another with a twisted ankle, and another with the flu. I would also act as an extra pair of hands with seriously ill, injured or violent patients. If things got hot and heavy with a disorderly patient, we could call for help and a bunch of people would be there instantly, unlike on the ambulance. I always tried to compliment the ambulance crews on their work with their patients—I knew where they were coming from, and positive feedback always went a long way.

I went to the waiting room one day to bring in a young male with "problems with his privates." I called his name and a tall, thin and boyish-looking young man stood up nervously and followed me. I did the usual ER admitting things, such as blood pressure, pulse, respiration rate, body temp and a brief history of the patient, including his major complaint. The major complaint was "sores" on his penis and he was obviously concerned that he had a sexually transmitted disease. I had him undress and get into a hospital gown.

I returned to the nursing station, finished writing up the chart and briefed Dr. Frank. She asked me to accompany her for the patient evaluation, so we went to the patient's cubicle. After some preliminaries, Dr. Frank asked to see the sores. He showed us some inflamed places around the head of his penis and Dr. Frank took a quick look and said she would be back shortly. I followed her out, and by the time we rounded the corner she was almost paralyzed with laughter. She looked at me and said, "Those are friction burns on his penis." That broke up the whole nurses' station and I blurted out, "What is the treatment? Play with something else?" Another nurse asked Dr. Frank, "Did you check his hands for friction burns too?"

Dr. Frank prescribed a cream to be put on the sores and advised complete abstinence for two weeks. I had to explain that this meant no sex and no masturbating. As I lingered on the words "no masturbating," I think he realized what the problem was, and he just nodded, grabbed the cream and discharge papers and left.

As I watched the embarrassed young man walk away, another patient rushed in and said that he had lopped off the tip of his finger. The index finger of his left hand was covered with duct tape, and I could see blood caked on the tape and oozing from beneath it. I grabbed his good arm and dragged him to the ER trauma room, then motioned to Holly for some help and we started to assess his injury. Apparently the guy worked in a sheet metal shop and he lost part of the finger in a cutter. This had happened at around quitting time and he had taped it back on so he could go drinking with his friends. I guess he thought the beer would kill the pain. But it didn't and his friends insisted he go to ER to get the finger reattached. To which our patient had replied that he had already reattached it, and "the hospital couldn't do no better."

The injury was not trivial: almost all of the fingernail and three quarters of an inch of the finger tip was severed. He had cut about halfway through the bone. He had no idea that reattaching a severed finger required plumbing in the vessels and wiring in the nerves and muscles. The finger was black and disgusting from hours of no blood flow, and there was no way to save it. He also lost out because we could not give him any strong painkillers because of the alcohol he had consumed. So he suffered for several hours while the alcohol wore off. His story made the papers with the headline, "Man Loses Finger and Finds a Bar."

In biology classes in college, we were learning about reproduction, which was always entertaining. In the ER, the male staff almost never tended to a female with gynecological problems, but the female staff would tend to males. Nonetheless, there were a few occasions when the male staff, myself included, would treat a female patient with a reproductive problem. On this day a Hispanic girl of about 16 came in complaining of stomach pain, nausea and vomiting for the past couple days. I asked as part of the standard workup if she was pregnant and she swore she was a virgin. Mary was a healthy teenager who lived in one of the overcrowded housing projects. After completing the general history and exam, I turned the information over to Dr. Frank. The doctor was a no-nonsense woman who had treated any number of pregnant females who assured her that their pregnancy was an immaculate conception. Dr. Frank did the usual procedures: a pelvic exam, blood test and a urine test to check for pregnancy and general health.

After the pregnancy test came back positive, Dr. Frank informed the staff that our Virgin Mary must have been a Mary Magdalene. None of us were surprised, and Dr. Frank went into the room to break the news. A few moments later, Dr. Frank scurried out of Mary's room to the coffee room, where she howled with laughter. Not wanting to miss a good story, the entire ER staff piled into the coffee room to hear what had transpired. Dr. Frank said, "After I told her she was pregnant, she continued to deny ever having sex. So I asked her what the sleeping arrangements were at home. She told me that she slept with her older sister and her sister's new husband. She also said that her sister and her husband were trying to make a baby." Dr. Frank now started to giggle. "Then she got a strange expression on her face and said with the greatest sincerity, 'Do you think I got splashed?'"

That was pretty much the end of the story, because Dr. Frank couldn't look at the poor girl without laughing. We had to call social services to assist the pregnant teen and the whole ER staff had a great time trying to explain to social services why we could not help "Virgin Mary Magdalene."

When I was not working in the ER or on the ambulance, I had to do my college work. I would often work in the university at night and even took occasional naps on the lab benches. Often the cleaning lady would come in and find me laid out on the lab table like a corpse. This startled the poor woman at first, and she claimed it nearly gave her a heart attack. Then she softened and said she felt guilty for waking me because it was evident that I needed the sleep. She was correct, because I never seemed to miss a night shift and was always sleep deprived.

During one night shift in the ER, I went to the waiting room to bring back a woman who had cut her hand while doing dishes. Apparently she'd had a dinner party, had a bit too much to drink, and cut her hand on a broken glass while trying to clean up. I went to the waiting room to fetch the name on my list and found out that the injured hostess was the cleaning lady from the university. (I hadn't known her name.) She was sitting next to her husband, clutching a bloody rag in her right hand. When she saw me she blurted out, "Wow, this is the first time I have ever seen you standing up!" Her husband looked at her and she quickly added, "I mean not laying down on a lab bench." Now the whole waiting room was aware of the dialogue and I was thoroughly embarrassed and so was she.

The husband started to laugh and said, "Is this the guy you always wake up at work?" The whole waiting room chuckled as I led the cleaning lady to the ER to get her hand sutured. I was only too happy to leave our audience.

When I started to work in the ER, I had already worked the ambulance for about six years, so I was pretty comfortable with most of the cases that rolled in. This led people to think that I was equally confident with all aspects of the job. But one job I was definitely not familiar with was putting catheters into male patients. A catheter is a tube that is placed up the urethra and into a person's bladder to drain urine. It was hospital policy that male staff members would catheterize male patients, and female staff looked after the female patients (although in practice, women sometimes did the procedure with males). During one night shift, the staff was short-handed and a male cancer patient in another part of the hospital required a catheter and they called on me. I had been shown the procedure only once, and had performed it (supervised) only once before. To make things worse, this patient had recently had prostate surgery, which would make passing a catheter very difficult and painful.

I talked to my patient to calm him down as well as myself. The staff immediately assumed I was an expert, unaware that this was my first solo performance. I went through the rituals of preparing the equipment and the area for the catheterization, as my patient watched intently. I draped sterile wrap over his penis and placed a doughnut-holed wrap around it. I then laid out another wrap under his penis and arranged some tubes and equipment that I would need, such as sterilizer and lubricant. With gloved hand I sterilized the tip of his penis and prepared it for the catheter. As I began to pass the catheter into his penis and up into his bladder, he took a deep breath and held it. I could feel the resistance this caused and could see the pain on his face. I eased the pressure on the tube and told him to inhale and exhale slowly and deeply. He did this, and it relaxed the muscles of his abdomen, which enabled me to pass the catheter into the bladder. Proud as I was, there were other patients to tend to, and I was off to other things.

As I finished the procedure he thanked me profusely. I pretended that it was all in a day's work, but I was just as relieved as he was. The two female nurses who had called me arrived to check on their patient. It was only then that they told me that they had tried to catheterize him twice before, but conceded that they needed an expert. If they only knew!

I would be called to the rescue again that night. Tom brought in a man who was unconscious from respiratory arrest, with the help of a police officer who had been driving the ambulance. The patient was Tom's partner. We got no advance notice of their arrival, because the driver generally calls the hospital while the person tending to the patient is busy in back, but the PO did not know how to do this.

Tom was ventilating his patient as he briefed us on what had happened. His partner was a new guy who had found that the building next to the ambulance garage sold and stored medical gases, including nitrous oxide or laughing gas. Tom's enterprising partner "borrowed" a tank of nitrous oxide and used the oxygen tubing from the ambulance to inhale it. He had made sure he would be able to breathe the nitrous oxide by taping a mask to his face. He'd done such a good job that he had become anoxic and gone into respiratory arrest.

Tom found his partner unconscious and unresponsive in the back of the ambulance, still connected by the tubing to the tank of laughing gas. To save his partner, Tom had to intubate the guy, wake up one of the cops in the bunkroom and rush to the ER, where we stabilized him and did some tests. The patient's blood gases were not good and there was no way that Tom was going to get his partner working again that night. This would mean the loss of ambulance service for the area. We could call mutual aid to get help from a neighboring town's ambulance, but that could take a long time. I was an obvious choice to work with Tom, and one of the senior nurses pointed out that historically the hospital ER had staffed the ambulance anyway. So there was precedent. It was agreed that Tom and I would work in the ER and respond to any ambulance calls that came in.

Tom's partner had to be admitted to the hospital over-night because of the risk of brain damage from the anoxia. He was eventually questioned by the police (for stealing the nitrous oxide) and thoroughly grilled by the ambulance administration as well. Because he was a new guy, he was told that he would not be let off probation and he voluntarily quit the ambulance a few weeks later. I made out very well that night, however, because the hospital paid me for the full shift that I was scheduled to work, *and* the ambulance paid me for the half shift I worked with Tom. All the money went to pay for my chemistry classes. We were learning about nitrogen gas exchange in plants and animals, something that Tom's partner should have been learning, too.

Spic and Span

I arrived on time for my shift one day and found that the ambulance and my partner for the night, John DeAngelo, were not there. The rig was out on a call, but a company supervisor, Jim Conner, was there as well as two other ambulances. Jim, not normally visible to the night-shift workers, had stayed late to do some paperwork. We met outside the call room, exchanged some pleasantries and went about our business. I went to the TV room and settled in to wait for John and my ambulance to arrive.

"What are you doing?" Jim asked me before I had a chance to turn the channel.

"Waiting for the rig to get back" was my answer.

"What about those rigs?"

"They're not mine."

"Well, I want you to detail them. They've been running all day and they're filthy. I want them spic and span, inside and out."

Jim was a typical supervisor. He hated to see an employee doing nothing. So I spent about 40 minutes detailing the two rigs to Jim's specifications. Two minutes after I finished, the crew with my rig returned and John DeAngelo was with them. Apparently, he had arrived early and went with them as a third man. Much to my chagrin, their ambulance was filthy, too, but we didn't have time to clean it, nor the authorization to use one of the ambulances that I had just detailed. So in a pretty grubby ambulance, John and I went to our first call.

John was relatively new on the job and anxious to help people. He really wanted to please those around him, including patients and co-workers. John was born in Puerto Rico and had a strong Hispanic accent. He was also fiercely proud of his heritage and defended all things Puerto Rican as being the best.

The shift was full of typical Friday night calls: drunks who fell down, drunks who got in a fight, nothing special or unusual, but John was always glad to help all those poor drunks. At 1:23 a.m. we got a call for a man stabbed in a bar fight. John drove to the address, a rough bar known for vicious fights, while I tried to not think about how disgusting our dashboard was compared to the ones I had cleaned.

We arrived at the bar and to my surprise only one police car was there. Normally a whole slew of cops would be dispatched for a bar fight with a stabbing.

We went in to find a very drunk, very large white male
with a switchblade knife sticking out of the middle of
the left forearm. The victim's name was Jerry, and he
was sitting on a bar stool, holding his injured arm palm
up on the bar, with his right hand pressing down on it.
The blade was sticking out between the fingers of his
right hand, which tightly gripped his left arm to slow
the bleeding. There was a pool of blood around his
left arm and one cop was taking notes from the victim.
I assumed other cops had already been there and left
with a suspect. I realized I was wrong about that when
Ron the cop turned to us and said, "Mr. Tough Guy
here wanted to prove he was tougher than anybody else
in the bar. So he pulls out a knife and impales his arm.
The knife goes completely though his arm and is stuck
into the wood of the bar."

There was a silence as we all stared at Jerry.

Ron went on. "Oh yeah, I forgot to say that Mr. Tough
Guy won't let me look at the arm because it hurts too
much to move it."

"OK, Jerry," I said, "I need to look at your arm." I
went to the patient and John broke out some bandages.

"Jerry, I want you to keep your right hand exactly
where it is. I am going to check the pulse of your
left hand. This shouldn't hurt, but tell me if it does.
Remember, just tell me it hurts—don't move or do
anything."

Since Jerry's left hand was palm up, it was easy to take
his pulse, which was strong, but rapid. I touched each of

Jerry's fingers to make sure that he had feeling in them, and he did. I told John that our patient had intact senses and distal pulses. Jerry was lucky, because he seemed to have no damaged nerves or arteries. The blade of the knife was parallel to the edge of his arm, so it probably passed between the two arm bones, the radius and ulna. There was less than a cup of blood loss and Jerry did not show signs of losing consciousness. The question was, how would we get him out of here?

The bar top was solid oak and much too thick to cut. I decided to apply pressure to the wound, secure the blade and handle to Jerry's arm with a bandage, and cut the tip of the knife off with a hacksaw.

"No, no, no!" screamed Jerry, "this is my favorite knife. You absolutely cannot cut the blade."

"Listen, Jerry, I am *not* pulling that knife out of your arm, and we have to get you to the hospital. Will you let me try to work the knife out of the wood? Before we do anything, we'll bandage your arm to keep it from hurting. Is that OK?"

"OK."

"Here is what we're going to do. John and I will wrap your arm and the knife together as one unit, and then we'll work it out of the bar. If it hurts too much, or if you start to bleed, we cut the knife, no argument. Deal?"

"Deal."

John and I bandaged the arm and secured the knife. When we were done we gently rocked the arm-plus-knife forwards and backwards to get the blade out of the wood. It finally pulled free—a little more than half an inch of knife blade had been stuck in the bar. We covered the tip of the knife with gauze and brought Jerry to the ED. Our next call came in as we were transferring Jerry to the ED stretcher. Just then, some intard started criticizing us for the large amount of bandages on Jerry's arm, because removing them would take a lot of time. I didn't have the chance to explain, so we left it to Jerry to tell the story. By the time we left, he was still trying to get assurances from the ED staff that the knife would not be damaged by them. The irony was that the cop told me the knife would be confiscated in any case, because Jerry had threatened people with it and used it as a weapon. This, I was sure, would bring Mr. Tough Guy to tears.

The next call was at a private home. In the bathroom we found an elderly man named Mark who had started to bleed profusely from his rectum. His wife met us at the door and brought us to Mark, who was naked, face down, with blood and feces still bubbling from his inflamed rectum.

His wife bent down to tell him we were there and try to comfort him. It was obvious from the mess on the floor that she was not only very worried about her husband's plight, but had vomited from the sight and smell. We dealt with the situation and got Mark to the hospital as fast as possible. He had lost a lot of fluids and needed to be treated quickly. At the hospital I worked on the paperwork of the two previous calls, while John cleaned the stretcher and the back of the ambulance of blood, feces and vomit.

The fetid slurry that Mark produced had overflowed onto the sheets, mattress and metal frame of the stretcher. John had done a pretty good job of cleaning things up, but the stretcher still smelled. The mattress was rubberized to make cleanup easier, but there was obvious discoloration in the stitching of the seams of the stretcher. So, you might say it was sort of clean*ish*.

John, always wanting to please, asked, "So what do you think? Clean?"

"Yeah, it's OK. It's spic and span*ish*," I quipped

The eager expression on John's face immediately soured.

"What do you mean *Spanish*? You don't like the way I talk? You calling me a Spic? What you saying, man?" John's voice revealed his obvious agitation.

John had seriously misunderstood what I was trying to say. I tried to explain my meaning to him. He claimed to have never heard the expression "spic and span," nor had he ever heard the suffix *-ish* used for "approximately." He truly thought I had made a racial slur. He spent much of the rest of the shift asking people what spic and span meant and or what *-ish* means at the end of a word. His attitude softened when people concurred with my definitions, but he didn't ever fully get over my comment.

John, if you read this, I wish I had said the stretcher was "pretty clean."

My Ambulance Ride

It is well established that doctors make terrible patients. That observation holds true for ambulance personnel as well.

I was on a family vacation at a lake in the mountains, a great way to relax and escape from the stress and tragedy of the streets. We were on the lake most of the day taking turns waterskiing, swimming, tubing and fishing. My passion was skiing. Fast slalom skiing on a hot summer day over a smooth shimmering lake is a feeling like no other. The goal of slalom skiing for me is to produce as much water spray as possible while cutting and jumping. A cut and jump on water-skis means zigzagging across the wake of the boat as fast as possible. When you reach the far side of the wake, you turn fast and go back across the wake. With practice, I was able to jump completely across the wake and splash on the other side, recover and do it all over again. I was having a great run, and I hit the boat wake for the best jump ever. When I cleared the wake this time, however, I nearly lost it and had to fight to keep my balance. The spray shooting up nearly blinded me, and when I regained control and could see clearly again, what I saw was a big red boat right in front of me. I was about to crash into an idling motorboat.

I remember very little of what I am about to describe; I am just reporting what people told me. Witnesses said that I tried to cut behind the boat, but only managed to hit closer to the idling engine and propeller. I passed under the boat and popped up on the other side, face down, unconscious and bleeding from the head.

After being pulled from the lake, bleeding and coughing up water, I was placed in the motorboat that I had hit. None of the bystanders were medically trained, so they drove me to the shore and moved me, without cervical support, onto the dock. Apparently someone on the beach saw the collision and had called 911. The driver of the motorboat found scalp and hair imbedded in the cracked fiberglass hull of his boat and decided to return it to me on the dock. The thought of a bloody tuft of skin and hair being laid on my chest while I was unconscious is a mental image that still makes me laugh, though no one was laughing at the time.

My father came on the scene, and although he is not medically trained, he was well aware that I was in danger. About this time, I regained partial consciousness and tried to comfort him by saying that I was all right, that this was no worse than getting my bell rung in a football game. I tried to get up and convince the family and bystanders that I was OK, but lapsed back to unconsciousness. The ambulance arrived and, briefly conscious again, I tried to tell them that I didn't need a backboard and that I could feel and move all my extremities. When I tried to demonstrate this by moving my left arm, however, a searing pain up my left arm and shoulder made me shout out in pain, as my arm refused to move.

The local Jolly Volly guys asked me what I could remember, and I said I remembered getting hit in the volleyball game. That was the wrong answer.

I was soon immobilized on a backboard, something I had done to hundreds of people, and loaded into the ambulance. I am told that I complimented the Jolly Vollys on how snug the immobilization was, because I couldn't move my head or shake it from side to side. They, of course, kept telling me to lie still, as they were concerned that I might have a neck injury.

When the ambulance guys passed me off to the ER doc, I remember correcting them by saying, "No I wasn't skiing, I was playing volleyball." My father tells me that I was conscious but not too coherent during my stay in the emergency room. I was admitted for observation overnight and discharged the next day with a huge headache.

I had spent thousands of hours working in an ambulance by that time, and now I had spent a short time in the back as a patient. I remember very little of it, which is probably a good thing, since I was not the best patient. But the experience did give me some insight on how the patients felt when we were treating and transporting them. I was amazed, for example, at how quickly everything changed. I went from skiing to being rescued in the water, to the ambulance, to the ER, to x-ray, to a hospital bed in just a few hours. In principle, I knew what was happening through all those steps, but it was still a whirlwind.

I was not in a lot of pain, and I was not afraid. Confused is what I mostly felt. It is common for a patient with a head injury to be not just confused but combative. It's not known why people with head injuries can get violent, but we had to take it into account when trying to treat the patient. This means soft restraints, talking a lot to the patient to keep him or her distracted, and ignoring bizarre behavior. The bizarre behavior, however, can make it difficult to assess the person's injuries, because they rarely give straight answers to investigative questions. While I was not combative, I kept telling the emergency personnel that I was OK and could move all my extremities. This was actually not the right thing for me to do, because I was at risk of a neck injury and such movements could further injure me. Even though I knew better, I did it anyway.

I learned some valuable lessons that day. I suddenly understood the seemingly irrational things my patients often did. I understood that a patient's aggressive or otherwise inappropriate behavior might be a sign of his or her illness or injury. I tried very hard from that point on to better understand the confusion and fear they were exeperiencing.

Holly Holiday

I was pulling some overtime after an overnight shift.
The shift had been busier than usual, and we hadn't
had a minute to have a meal or do the paperwork.
My partner had gone home to the wife and kids and
I stayed to write up the numerous calls of the day.
Amazingly, even with notes from a call eight or 10
hours earlier, it was sometimes hard to remember the
details. I really disliked backloading the run sheets this
way, but sometimes it had to be done, and today was
such a day.

I was camped out in the quiet room of the ED so that
I could sneak a peek at the charts of our patients if I
needed some forgotten details, such as the name of a
patient. None of the calls were remarkable in any way,
but the shift's run sheets looked like a shopping list of
grief: car accident with one dead and one unconscious;
elderly woman fell down and broke her hip; suspected
heart attack with shortness of breath; elderly husband
whose wife could not wake him up (and never would).

The list went on and on in an expanding blur. This was pretty depressing. I still wanted to help people and today I seemed to have helped no one.

I was engrossed in describing the events of the day when Holly walked in—in tears. At first I thought someone had died and she was a relative coming to the quiet room to grieve. But it really was Holly with tears streaming down her face. I had barely been able to ask what was wrong when she blurted out the answer.

"I'm moving," she said.

"When?"

"This weekend."

She went on to explain that her mother was an alcoholic and her family was moving near a rehab center in Omaha, Nebraska. Holly was going to transfer to a nursing school there. Apparently the family had been trying to get out of the city for a while and an opportunity had finally come up, but it had to be seized immediately. It sounded as if the rehab center was like a country club for subabs. Although Holly was an adult and could stay or live wherever she wanted, her two younger sisters could not be unsupervised (their father had died over a decade ago), and Holly had to stay with them.

Omaha was a long way away, and the weekend was only three days from now. I was gutted and speechless at the thought of losing of Holly and equally distressed by the knowledge that things had been so difficult for her at home. She had never told me about any of this.

 "Will I be able to see you before you go?" I asked.

"Well, I have some things to finish up here and also need to help my sisters get packed. I don't have much free time."

Without any prompting from me, Holly started to confide in me.

"When I was younger, I thought I would be in control of my life. I wanted to escape our grim life with Mom and her drinking and take care of people. My father died of a heart attack and better medical care might have saved him. So I decided to become a nurse. I really want to care for people. I was good at it with my sisters, and even with my mother when she was completely out of it.

"Now here I am, an adult, but I can't get out from under my mother's addiction to alcohol. People say that alcoholism is a disease. I don't believe that. My mother hides behind the word 'disease' by saying she is sick, and that because I am a nurse I should take care of her. Calling it a disease gives her an excuse, like it's *not* her fault. She wants a pill to get better and a handicapped sticker on the car so she can park close to the liquor store. All because she thinks she has a disease. I think it's a behavior. And like anyone who misbehaves, she should be punished. But she's not, and she takes none of the responsibility. Meanwhile, I'm punished because I am the child of an alcoholic. This is so unfair. Life is so unfair."

Holly stopped crying and went on in an almost clinical tone. "I was working in hospice today, caring for a woman about my mother's age. She will die of cancer soon, and her family is there constantly and they all love and support her. *She* is dying of a disease. *She* should get a pill or a treatment to get better. But there is none. I actually wished it was my mother who was dying and not this woman. My mother seems to have neglected everything in her life except the bottle, and this woman who has not just herself, but everyone around her to live for will not survive for long. I couldn't even count all the chances we have given my mother, and here we are giving her another one. Why can't the woman in the hospice get a second chance? Mom's on her millionth chance."

Holly's words and emotion hung heavy in the air. I stared at her. "I love you, Holly," is what I wanted to say, but all I said was, "Is there anything I can do?"

"No. Thanks for listening. You obviously have work to do, and I've talked your ear off. I should let you go. I hope to see you before I go. I'll let you know my new address when I find out what it is. If you want to write or visit, that is."

"Yes, please make sure you give me your address. I can actually write things that are not run sheets. You might be surprised."

With that she smiled and left.

The Big One

Training for the Big One is an integral part of any city EMS procedure. The term refers to a major disaster that involves police, fire department, ambulance, hospital and morgue. I participated in disaster drills in two different cities. One took place when I was working in the emergency room. The ER staff was instructed to break out the supplies, set up the spare stretchers and stock several storerooms to be used as patient rooms. We were then assigned to the mock patients as they were wheeled in, generally one physician and one nurse to each seriously injured patient. This worked well, and we went through mock treatments of the patients and shifted them to the floors or to the operating room. Prior to the drill, the hospital and EMS made sure that there was extra staff available. This was done to ensure that the real patients were not neglected while key staff got practice in the procedures of the drill. The second disaster drill I participated in was more unexpected.

Tom and I were working a 7 a.m. to 7 p.m. shift, and around noon I was looking for Holly, but couldn't find her. No one had seen her and I couldn't find any of the other nursing students to ask. Just then we were dispatched to a bleacher collapse at the high school stadium. On the EMS radio, we could hear that the fire department had been called too. This sounded like the Big One. Excitedly we raced to the scene. When we arrived, there was an official-looking guy with a red cross on his chest, holding a clipboard. He flagged us down and said, "This is the city disaster drill." Tom and I had no prior knowledge of this, so we were a bit confused. The Red Cross guy went on. "Park your ambulance over there and use this disaster equipment to work the drill. Your calls will be covered by pre-arranged mutual aid."

I was the first senior EMS person there, so according to SOP, I was the triage officer for the scene. Tom and I parked the ambulance as instructed and brought the equipment over to the scene. It appeared that the bleachers were in the process of repair, and patients in makeup were spread all around them. This included people supposedly impaled on some of the structures and a wide range of other trauma.

As the triage officer I evaluated the injuries of each patient I came across. I had a stack of colored tags that represented the different priorities. Tom did immediate care based on how I assessed the patients. He then turned our patients over to the fire department and other EMS people who were following us.

Several of the patients (many of whom were nursing students) were "walking wounded," and I asked them to go to the tent that was set up for on-scene treatments. The assessment of the patients was done in two ways. The walking wounded were usually made up to have injuries like a broken arm or cut face, and I could talk to them. Other patients were lying on the ground with a little card that said something like "unconscious or unable to respond" and had a brief summary of vitals. Many of these patients had what looked like professional makeup to represent various injuries. During my previous training I had become familiar with these makeup techniques and mock injuries.

Tom and I came across a patient with a card on his chest and I saw a red tube going up his right arm. My experience told me that there was a mock arterial bleed coming: the tube in his arm was going to squirt blood at us. So I asked Tom to check the blood loss on that patient. Tom got the full effect of the arterial bleeding. He did a quick field dressing and turned the patient over to the EMS people behind us, who acted as transporters to take people to the hospital.

After tagging a bunch of other patients, I came across Holly. Tom said, "Oh no, your girlfriend looks pretty serious." After a pause he continued. "Now you're supposed to say, 'We all know she's pretty.'" Holly smiled at us, but could say nothing because her tag said she was DOA.

"It seems that you're dead. Can I still do mouth to mouth?" I asked her teasingly.

"You might be able to save me with some heart massage," she joked.

"I think I'll give you a black tag to keep you here for now, and come back and try some intensive physical therapy." Holly laughed.

Tom and I trolled through the rest of the patients at the scene, gave everyone their priority tag and went back to help care for the remaining victims. Happily, this led us back to Holly. She was still there amongst the prearranged debris of the bleachers with her gray makeup causing her to look like a real corpse.

"You know, I have never engaged in necrophilia, but in your case I would be willing to make an exception." She really laughed at that, and said, "I'm glad you guys came back, it was dead quiet here."

"Nice comeback for a corpse," I said. "'If we make it through this alive, can we still be friends?"

"Well, I don't know. I thought you might be my knight in shining armor and save me."

Before we could continue our innuendoes and clichés, a Red Cross guy ran over and advised Tom and I that mutual aid was busy and that we had a real call to go to. After wishing Holly a quick recovery from her recent death, Tom and I left for a car accident not far from the stadium. It didn't take long to get the victim stabilized and transferred to the ER. When we got there, I tried to see if Holly was in the makeshift morgue set up in the ER, but she was not. So much for being a knight in shining armor.

After Tom and I had written up the car accident, we joined the other medical personnel in the office to debrief on the drill. We talked about the number of patients involved and what had worked well, what might be improved, and so on. We patted each other on the back for a job well done. The consensus of both the administration and those who had worked the drill was that we were ready for the Big One.

A few weeks later, Tom and I were working a rainy Saturday afternoon when we heard on the radio that several police cars had been dispatched to a notoriously dangerous section of highway for an accident. An ambulance was not yet called. Tom and I listened hard for word from the police when they arrived on scene. Suddenly we heard the excited voice of one of the rookie cops. "Tractor-trailer truck, lots of cars, people screaming, lots of cars," he stuttered. The calm voice of the dispatcher now came on, "How many cars involved?"

"12," came the answer. Twelve cars and a tractor-trailer would mean a massive accident. This was serious. This could be the Big One.

The dispatcher immediately initiated the disaster response protocol. This meant dispatching police, ambulance, fire and emergency management people at the same time. Just as with the bleacher collapse, Tom and I were going to be the first ambulance on the scene. I drove as Tom was breaking out the disaster kit from the back. We could hear the fire department and mutual aid being called to the scene. The police were sending their mobile command center to take charge, and other police cars were sent to stop traffic from entering the six-lane highway from either direction.

Tom and I got to the scene just as two other police cars arrived. It was still raining, and we could see a car carrier on its side and several cars strewn around on the ground like a child's toys. But the cars were all from the carrier. The truck had been in an accident with another vehicle. The result was cars everywhere, but only one person was injured in the accident. The inexperienced cop had inadvertently caused a disaster drill to be initiated because of an MVA with one injury. Tom and I went to investigate the injuries in the one car that did have a driver, and we tried to avoid the confusion that was mounting around us as more and more people and equipment arrived. This was not the Big One, and for that we were thankful.

When I stopped working on the ambulance, I had never experienced the Big One, and I consider myself very lucky for that. When I heard about disasters like the Oklahoma City bombing and the tragedy of September 11, 2001, I have a special sympathy not only for the victims of these disasters, but the EMS personnel who work through events like these. These people are recognized as the heroes they are, but often they are victims too. Working the Big One does not leave EMS personnel untouched.

I had an opportunity to talk to Tom after he responded to a massive fire with 26 dead and more than 40 injured. As he related the story to me, I noticed his expressionless face. The blank stare in his eyes said to me he was a million miles away, still reliving the experience. Although his voice sounded dispassionate, I could sense the emotion grinding inside of him. He told me that he had to transport "a load of bodies," and that the head of one of the victims exploded, causing brain matter to ooze onto the stretcher and the floor of the ambulance. From his description, I knew what had happened was that the heat had become so intense that the victim's brain had expanded, causing the skull to break. Instead of expressing sadness or remorse at the loss of life, Tom could only muse at the mess of "cooked brain" he had to clean up. I never, ever heard him use the expression Big One after that.

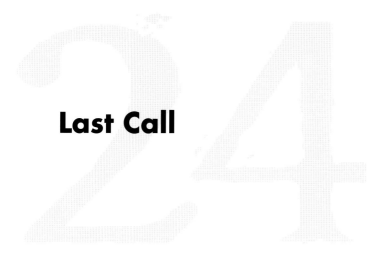

Last Call

People sometimes ask me why I quit the ambulance.
The answer is simple: I burned out. That always leads
to the next question, "How did you know you had
burned out?"

That story is hard to tell, but I need to try. It is a story
I am not proud of, and one I have avoided telling until
now, because it reminds me of the depths of cynicism
I had achieved. Recall that my goal upon joining the
ambulance was to help people, and while I strove to
achieve that, the heartache of life on the streets and on
the ambulance was too much to bear. College was a
respite from all of this, and for a while it gave me purpose. But I was having a harder and harder time keeping my college and ambulance lives separate. My cynicism was beginning to show itself in my studies.

Sometimes during the week, when I was not working on the ambulance, I would study in my dorm room. The room had lofts with the beds up high and desks underneath. We had set things up this way so that we had extra floor space. I would often hang blankets from my bed to make my own little study in the room. This was necessary because the room often would be a kind of meeting place. With practice, I would be able to study at my desk with people drinking and partying behind me.

One day when I was studying biochemistry, I heard a music major named Lisa come in and exclaim that Professor Kettering, the conductor for her upcoming classical concert, was an inconsiderate idiot. I tried to focus on the biochemistry of endorphins, where they signal changes in the body, but Lisa was loud. She was a gifted musician and sure she was destined for a great career as a performer. Generally I could filter out such noise, but Lisa's high-pitched voice made it hard to do so. She said Professor Kettering had the whole orchestra focus on practicing a certain piece and did not give her any time to practice her solo. She was furious at him for being insensitive to her needs as an artist, knowing it would be detrimental for her not to have an opportunity to perform her solo with the whole group. She went on and on, and eventually segued to bragging about how prestigious the solo was and how important it would be to have everyone appreciate her prowess on the violin. The length and depth of her diatribe was exhausting.

I tried again to focus on endorphins, the body's natural opiates. I had some experience with what opiates did, because they were the drug of choice for a lot of junkies. Opiates were in heroin, morphine and a lot of other street drugs, so I had seen their addictive and destructive effects. I tried to concentrate until the word "endorphin" started to look like "dolphin." About this time, Lisa drew me into her crisis.

"Joe, do you plan to come hear me at the concert, and don't you agree that the fair thing would have been for Kettering to have me work on my solo?"

"Well, no, I don't plan to go to the concert because I have to work." This caused a withering glance from Lisa. "What's the big deal with the concert, anyway?"

"What do you mean, 'big deal?'" she exclaimed indignantly. "It's a pivotal point of my career. There will be talent scouts at the concert, and I could be discovered. My goal in life is to be one of the greats, and this is only a start, but an important one. My success as a performer will actually benefit Professor Kettering, but he ignored my need to interact with the rest of the orchestra. Some of those freshmen have no timing and they have to learn my routine from me."

I still felt it was no big deal. A severed limb is a big deal. The day before I had to wash brain matter out of the cuffs of my shirt. That was a big deal. I couldn't stop myself from pushing on with the conversation.

"So what would you consider to be a crowning achievement for you in your career?"

"That's easy: a command performance at Carnegie Hall."

"So your overall goal in life is to have a large number of people tell you how great you are. Your whole life's ambition is all about you."

This made Lisa bristle. "No, you don't understand. I want to bring joy to people with my performances. My music makes people happy."

"If you wanted to bring joy to people with your music, you could be a street performer and bring joy to people passing by. There's no need for Carnegie Hall. You are all about having people fawn over you. If you look at things from the perspective of the greater good, maybe Kettering has it right in trying to bring the freshmen up to standard and let you, the virtuoso, do it yourself. Why don't you stay and practice here. That way I won't have to miss your performance."

Lisa left the room and I immediately regretted confronting her that way. She was an excellent musician, and I respected and admired her drive to be successful. Sometimes my life on the ambulance and my college life did not mix well, and this was one of those times. I went back to my chemistry text. The endorphins still looked like dolphins.

I wrote a brief letter to Holly, told her of my conversation with Lisa and tried to explain my position. I knew she would understand, because she had been on the job and experienced life in the streets. I was planning to visit Holly over the next summer vacation. For me it would be a vacation from the ambulance as well as from school.

A few days later—in fact, it was the day that Lisa was performing her solo—Bill and I were called to a private home at about three in the morning. The call came in simply as "woman is sick." We arrived there right behind a PO who was the younger sister of Richie, the dispatcher. This was a bad sign, because Richie was mad at his sister, so he was only sending her on bad calls. We were greeted at the door by a college-aged male who informed us his mother was vomiting blood. In the third-floor bedroom of this ancient brownstone, we found a heavy woman in her late 40s in white flannel pajamas. The room, bed and pajamas were covered with blood and vomit. The smell of vomit and the sickly sweet smell of alcohol permeated the room. I checked her pulse and tried to establish an airway. There was no pulse. Bill called for backup because the three of us were not going to be able to carry this woman down the stairs.

It was pretty clear to Bill and I what had happened. This woman was bleeding to death from her esophagus. Esophageal varices are inflamed veins in the esophagus, often caused by chronic alcoholism. This disease is made worse if the person has liver disease causing more swelling and pressure on the veins of the esophagus, and making the inflammation hard to heal and prone to bleeding. If the inflammation is bad enough, the person can bleed to death.

Although I was pretty sure what the answer would be I asked the question anyway. "Does she drink?"

"Well, when she drinks, she drinks," was the response from an older male in the room, probably her son. I noticed that there was a growing entourage of family members assembling from various places in the house.

I continued. "Does she have any medical conditions that might cause this?"

The college-aged male said, "Yeah, she has a very closed food tube."

The esophagus is the food tube, and "very closed" sounds a lot like varicose, so we had our diagnosis and prognosis. The survival rate for a patient who has bleeding esophageal varices is nearly zero, so she was probably going to die tonight. I had never heard of someone surviving ruptured esophageal varices. Physicians spend a lot of time preparing a family for the terrible and messy end in a case like this. The difficult conversations that physicians must have with their patients and their families are usually referred to as "breaking the bad news," and it is always difficult to be delicate and sensitive in such a discussion. The family should have known her diagnosis and have been fully aware that she was going to die from this. Still, we had two ambulance crews and a police officer working to try to save her. I continued to try to get an airway, but the clots were so thick and abundant that we burned out one suction unit and needed the other from the backup ambulance. We worked hard to keep her alive.

Even though we all knew that Mrs. Jefferson was likely to die that morning, we started two IVs on her, and the hospital transfused her when we arrived. The ER physician finally called the code and pronounced Mrs. Jefferson dead at 4:13 a.m. She died in the code room in the hospital (the same room where I had fallen asleep standing up) and now the ED doc needed to break it to the Jefferson family.

The ED had a special "quiet room" where physicians, social workers, and the like could meet with family and help them begin the grieving process. This was where the Jeffersons should get the bad news. The ER waiting room was choked with members of the Jefferson family, and we wanted to get them all to the quiet room. I suggested that they ask the college-age male, whose name was Tillis, to help get the family there. He seemed to understand, but insisted that the ER doc first tell him if his mother had survived, because "Ol' Doc Wilson said that the very closed thing would kill her." The ER doc informed him that his mother had indeed died and that it was best to tell the family in the quiet room. Nodding, Tillis marched to the waiting room where the Jefferson family was awaiting word. With all eyes on him, he announced, "Momma's dead."

With that the room broke down into hysterical shouting and denial. Most were saying it was not true, and that the incompetent ambulance people with bad equipment and an inefficient ER had killed her. How could they be accusing us of killing her from a disease she gave to herself over years of substance abuse? I truly felt that she had killed herself with the help and endorsement of her family while the emergency services and myself tried to save her. The wails and accusations and apparent surprise of the family, who knew her lethal diagnosis, echoed throughout the ED. The cacophony especially caught me by surprise because Tillis had seemed so calm and ready for it.

I didn't know how to act or what to do. Part of me wanted to laugh in the face of this family tragedy. I had worked hard to save someone we all knew was going to die and now I was being accused of murder. I actually had to stifle a laugh, and I rushed away from them before they saw me. Yet I also felt incredibly guilty at my insensitivity and cynicism.

At that moment, I knew that I had had enough of the ambulance. I was a burnout and it was time to leave.

AFTERWORD

The time I spent on the ambulance shaped and directed my professional career. It allowed me to complete a bachelor's degree in chemistry, a masters in biological sciences and a PhD in physiology. My research has recently revealed a new family of molecules that is present in the spinal fluid of patients who have suffered a stroke. I am now working to prove that these molecules cause about 10 percent of all strokes and, more important, to develop therapies to treat those patients. It is my sincere hope that my research will help thousands of people in the treatment and diagnosis of stroke. All this has come about because of decisions and events that occurred with Alice, Pinto, and other patients on the ambulance, as well as Dr. Daniels, Dr. Frank, and partners such as Bill, Tom, Richie and others. It is unfortunate that I eventually burned out, but that experience has made me almost obsessively determined to do research that will truly help people. That has always been my guiding principle.

GLOSSARY

AOB: alcohol on breath

ARP: a Puerto Rican gang member

Call jumping: racing to a scene to which another ambulance has been called

Code: a cardiac arrest and the associated procedures and treatments that are needed when a heart stops beating

Cop shop: police station

CPR: cardiopulmonary resuscitation

DMZ: demilitarized zone; in EMS jargon, a police station, because it held the fewest guns in the neighborhood

DOA: dead on arrival

ED: emergency department

ER: emergency room

EKG: electrocardiogram

EMS: emergency medical services

EMT: emergency medical technician

ETA: estimated time of arrival

FD: fire department

FNG: fucking new guy

getting soft: removing sharp or dangerous equipment (pens, etc.) from your pockets before dealing with a dangerous patient

GSW: gunshot wound.

intard: an intern with no idea what he or she is doing

IV: intravenous (i.e. fluids injected into a vein)

Homme: (pronounced "homey") a black gang member

Jolly Volly: volunteer ambulance

kissing Ethyl: drinking alcohol

KON: knock on the nut, i.e. a head injury

LAC: laceration

LOC: loss of consciousness

LOL: little old lady

ME: medical examiner

MPI: multiple personal injuries

mutual aid: an agreement whereby emergency services from a neighboring area can be called upon to help when necessary

MVA: motor vehicle accident

Narcan: a trade name for the drug naloxone, given to overdose victims to counteract the effects of heroin and other narcotics

NAD: no apparent distress

no-man's land: low-income housing projects, or the protected turf of any gang

OD: overdose

PI: personal injury

PFN: plain fucking nuts

proby: a new employee on probation

Quinlaned: overdosed on alcohol and drugs

rig: ambulance

rose garden: the terminal unit in a hospital, normally used for severely brain damaged patients

SOB: short(ness) of breath

SOP: standard operating procedure

subab: substance abuser

tattooing: the carving of gang insignias on the face or chest of a rival gang member

tunnel vision: the tendency for an EMS person to focus solely on the patient without being aware of their surroundings, especially dangerous conditions around them

WT: a white gang member

ABOUT THE AUTHOR

Joseph F. Clark has lived in Oxford, Paris and Moscow, and now resides in Cincinnati with his partner Janice and their 10 cats. He is currently a scientist and researcher at the University of Cincinnati, studying the causes and treatments of stroke.

Joe has authored or co-authored more than 70 scientific journal articles and three scientific texts.

PICTURE CREDITS

Every effort has been made to obtain permissions for the images used in this book. If there have been errors or omissions, please contact Firefly Books, and we will amend these credits in future printings.

Page 129: Bea Clark; Bob Smith
Page 130: Joe Clark; Bob Smith
Page 131: Bob Smith; Bob Smith
Page 132: Joe Clark; Joe Clark
Page 133: Joe Clark; Jim Clark
Page 134: Bob Smith; Bob Smith
Page 135: Bob Smith; Bob Smith
Page 136: Bob Smith; Daniel Davenport, University of Cincinnati Academic Health Center Communications Services

INDEX

ambulance responses to
  broken bones
    arm 195
    jaw 171-173
  burns 17-20
  carbon monoxide poisoning 12-14
  cardiac arrest 32-33, 109-111, 141-142, 184-185
  chemical ingestion 44-45
  congestion 151-153
  crushed limbs 59-61
  epilepsy 148-149
  falls 16-17, 42-43, 170-171, 193-194
  gunshot wounds 14-16, 48-50, 100-102, 121, 162-163
  head injuries 111-114
  insulin comas 33-35
  labor pains 164
  lacerations
    from broken glass 173-174
    from cutting wrists 45-47
    from knife wounds 21-24, 218-221
    from physical fights 167-170
  nerve damage 25-26
  psychotic behavior 36-40, 190-192
  rectal bleeding 221-222
  ruptured esophageal varices 243-246
  seizure 187-188
  severed hand 83-88
  stroke 88-91
  struck pedestrian 73-75, 77-79, 144-146, 149-150
  tattooing, forceful 96-98
  vehicular accidents 11, 32, 52-59, 61-62, 64-72,
    75-77, 114-116, 123-128, 179-180, 235-236

Clark, Joseph F.
  his medical education and training 8-10, 25-27, 52,
    55, 82, 91, 103-105, 157-159, 182-183, 212, 226,
    231-235, 239-242
  his own hospitalization 223-226
  his ultimate burnout 243-246
communication 99-100
coping mechanisms
  alcohol 96, 162
  compartmentalizing 95-96
  humor 13-17, 19, 24, 54, 63-64, 72, 95-96, 116, 160
  justification, religious and other 96, 160
  visiting newborns 161, 163-165
debilitating injuries 203-206
drug users 62, 119-128, 149-150, 154-157
drunks 32, 148, 167-176
emergency room responses to
  catheters, need for insertion of 213-214
  friction burns 208-209
  gunshot wounds 199-200
  pregnancies 210-211
  respiratory arrests 214-215
  severed fingers 209-210
heart attack *see* cardiac arrest
holidays 11, 29-35
Kissler Rehabilitation Institute 203-205
occupational hazards
  blood-born diseases 97-98
  dangerous surroundings 53, 65, 188-190
  emotional stress 23-24, 157, 176, 237
  incorrect procedures 184-185
  noxious substances 85-87, 110-114, 221-222

sleep deprivation 93-94, 96, 101-105, 207, 212
vehicle malfunction 120
violence 99, 120-121, 123-128, 153-157, 159,
    162-163, 174-176, 181-183
public interference
    disruptive onlookers 42-43, 65-67, 115-116, 188-189
    obstructing emergency personnel 137-139
    tailgating ambulance 141-142
Quinlane, Karen Ann 47
Quinlaned 47-48, 63
Red Cross 232-235
suicide 21-24, 41-43, 45-50, 77-79
tunnel vision 73-80, 180-181